Warrior Angel

Warrior Angel

Beyond Disability: A Family's Quest for Ordinary

by Susan Dunnigan

Warrior Angel

Celticfrog Publishing, Kamloops, BC

© 2020 Susan Dunnigan

Excerpt from "Homage to Rosengarten" from *The Flame: Poems, Notebooks, Lyrics, Drawings* by Leonard Cohen. Copyright © 2018 by Old Ideas, LLC. Reprinted by permission of Farrar, Straus and Giroux for the world not including the Commonwealth.

Extracts from "Homage to Rosengarten" from *The Flame: Poems and Selections from Notebooks*, reproduced by permission of Canongate Books Ltd in Canada and for the Commonwealth used by permission of The Wylie Agency LLC

ISBN: 978-1-989092-48-4

Design and cover art by Neil Dunnigan and Kate James.

Sculpture depicted on the cover created by artist Dan Friesen.

Printed by Ingram Spark.

Dedication

This book is dedicated to Matthew James Dunnigan, with love. A son, brother, uncle, cousin, friend and citizen, his life journey illuminates key lessons about humanity, capacity, resilience and self-determination.

With unwavering support from family and allies, Matthew bravely ventures beyond the confines of disability, striving to tap his potential as an ordinary citizen. Walking the journey at Matthew's side has challenged, enriched and strengthened every family member, undeniably making us better human beings.

Matthew's generosity of spirit and maturity, like his father's and sister's, far outweighed the discomfort of revealing in this book the full spectrum of indelible memories and potent life lessons. Our family's quest for "ordinary" has been unpredictable, heart-warming, gut-wrenching and never boring. In short, one hell of a ride, but well worth the price of admission: unconditional love.

And here She is:

Fully born from herself

Urgent and accommodating

A thrust of polished energy that does not cut the air

But softens it and ignites it softly

—Leonard Cohen, "Homage to Rosengarten"

from The Flame: Poems and Selections from Notebooks,

McClelland & Stewart, 2018

Table of Contents

Foreword

By Michael Kendrick, PhD
Kendrick Consulting International

Whoever attempts to describe a person's life is faced with the challenge of understanding how that person's soul has defined their life and how the decisions they have made have shaped, and reflect, the soul's journey. As Susan shares early in this book about her son Matthew, "his life journey illuminates key lessons about humanity, capacity, resilience and self-determination." The lives of most people are usually not captured by a book describing their journey.

This is especially the case with people who much of society may scarcely notice or see value in because of their disabilities or some other perceived difference. Yet, matters of great significance may nonetheless manifest in all lives, whether appreciated by others or even by themselves. Matthew's mother, in writing this book, has demonstrated admirable respect for his journey by trying to name and capture its importance and significance.

Matthew not only has lived robustly despite his disabilities; his life has been probed for meaning and significance by himself and by others. His mother, in both writing about and being a participant, has not just described his life, she has also sought to better comprehend the layers, directions and significance of experiences and their possible deeper meanings. We might all be honoured were someone to do the same for us. Yet, at the same time, many of us might find ourselves concerned about the likelihood that others might not see us at our best. For Matthew's mother, the urge to protect her child and his image in the minds of others necessarily coexists with the need to tell his life story accurately.

This book is driven by Matthew's family's urgent desire that he access the richness of an "ordinary life." Their arduous quest nurtured his full citizenship, beyond the narrow confines of being protected and "safe," sidelined at the margins of human potential. In explaining her family's highest intent, Susan states that "nurturing a warrior angel spirit increases the odds of a vulnerable person thriving—not just surviving—in life." Thus, this book is about the family's cultivation of a "warrior angel spirit" in themselves, Matthew and his other allies, so that Matthew might flourish. There was a time when there were hardly any books written about the lives of persons with disabilities, as many people might have rarely encountered such persons in their everyday lives. People with all manner of disabilities have existed outside of or at the margins of society throughout much of known human history. Many were hidden from view, often in remote residential institutions, rarely venturing into the mainstream pathways of community life.

Through more than a century of visionary leadership by many persons with disabilities, we have witnessed a gradual liberation of people with disabilities to truer and much fuller versions of themselves. This self-advocacy has been given greater momentum by the simultaneous advocacy of families, human service professionals, academics, politicians and public servants for similarly positive visions of what life could become for people with disabilities.

When we have been open to exploring a vision of "what could be" rather than "just what is now," we have seeded revolutions again and again in the kinds of bountiful lives people with disabilities can and should experience. Susan proactively integrated her knowledge, skills and passion as a parent, advocate and professional to positively influence Alberta's disability policy and practice. Like many others, she has been part of mobilizing a social movement for change, so that Matthew and countless others might be more fully engaged in community. That change in ever-expanding opportunities has gradually come about and has continued to evolve. In this book, Susan has accomplished naming and embodying this spiritual quality that ultimately leads to progress— that is, the spiritual ethic that cultivates "warrior angels."

The positive news for Matthew and many others is that he was enabled, notwithstanding the challenges of living with a disability, to access a wide range of normal and appealing opportunities entirely within community. Typically, these opportunities were the same as those of most people his age and generation. For Matthew, many societal enticements brought with them potential trials and tribulations that can face anyone in their search for fulfillment. This sense of having to manage the many hazards embedded in seemingly ordinary community living also applied to his parents, as they tried to support Matthew through life's unpredictability. His mother describes his parents' experience, and that of his sister, as often being a "high-wire act." Chapter after chapter, we see a recurring need for "striking the balance" so that Matthew could have the decent life that both he and his family sought for him.

Of course, often the risk is not quite striking the balance in a satisfying way. Matthew was as burdened as his parents were in "getting the balance right." He naturally had his own priorities and life purposes and acted on them with the same determination seen in his family. Matthew himself contributed to these struggles in how he managed himself, his decisions and his responsibilities. As Edith Hamilton said in her 1964 book, *The Ever-Present Past*, "responsibility is the price every person must pay for freedom." Matthew had both freedoms and responsibilities to contend with as he grew and developed as a person.

Both the advances and setbacks for Matthew in the ongoing struggle to realize his potential and to find his best path through life have often been demanding, costly, distressing and inescapable in terms of unsought consequences, frustrations and disappointments. Ingrained in the pursuit of an ordinary life, these elements contributed to his personal growth, wisdom and maturity. In supporting Matthew's will for self-direction, his family and others have repeatedly had to be part of managing whatever has ensued.

Consequently, while this book clearly chronicles Matthew's story, it is also the story of the other people in his life and their many contributions and challenges along the way. Matthew's journey has been intertwined with a large number of people's lives, of which only some are highlighted in the book. Advocates for people with disabilities, including parents and their allies, have long promoted normal community living for persons with disabilities. Not surprisingly, Matthew has lived within the broad community with all of the positive and negative aspects that come with it. Without romanticizing community life or questioning its benefits, this book adds a very valuable and granular sense of realism about the hardships and risks that are intertwined with the jewels. Matthew's life has not always been easy and successful, nor has it been that way for his family, friends and other allies in their support of Matthew. Notably, Matthew's journey has nevertheless been marked by boundless possibilities and wonder. The life lessons learned by Matthew and previously described by his mother as "*humanity, capacity, resilience and self-determination*" are not lessons solely for Matthew, but for all people as they seek their own meaningful life and find themselves lifted up, challenged and grateful for their own "warrior angels." Consequently, the reader will not be disappointed in moving through the inherent drama of an interesting life well lived, as these kinds of fundamental life challenges will resonate. Not only is Matthew's life enriched, but also the lives of his family, allies and diverse companions along the way.

The book reads well, as each chapter cumulatively adds to the breadth and depth of Matthew's journey. Each includes many surprises, meanings, and much growth, so that by the time the reader gets to the end, they realize anew just how much drama and interest can be contained in everyday life moments and incidents. That sense is added to by the mounting discovery of just how intriguing Matthew and the people around him turn out to be. Matthew's disability rapidly recedes as a pertinent factor for the reader as they become progressively drawn into the many dramas and events of his life. What engages us is his personality, spirit and management of his life and how they shape the lives of the many people and events in his life.

The quote "may you live in interesting times" was first used by Sir Austen Chamberlain in 1936, and later popularized through a speech by Robert F. Kennedy in 1966. Many have said that the phrase is a curse that originated in ancient Chinese times, whereas others have seen it as representing the existential wholeness of life itself—that is, that life can be both a blessing and a curse at times. Certainly, if one were to pick any of the days portrayed in Matthew's journey, one might quite regularly find one's share of blessings and curses.

In a larger sense, we all are a blessing or a curse potentially to and for others, much as others are that for us at times. The "good life" was never meant to be without hardships or difficulties, or we would not grow, learn, develop or thrive. Matthew's life has had its share of struggles and adversity, but the reader will soon discover that it has also, more often than not, been the life that those who love Matthew had so rightly wanted for him. What should not be lost from sight, nonetheless, is that a key part of a fulfilling life is the person themself setting their own course. There is no doubt after reading this book that Matthew has set his own course throughout his life and that is a key "good" in "the good life."

Acknowledgements

Multiple people encouraged, mentored and supported me during every phase of creating this book, from concept to completion. Their diverse gifts, strong spirits and quiet strength all influenced the project, some briefly and some for the duration. Within this eclectic group, particular individuals stand out and were essential to this book becoming a reality.

I have been fortunate to accumulate a broad network of allies who share my passion for community inclusion. Garnered over decades, the spectrum includes family, friends, kindred spirits and professionals. While not all are mentioned in the book, be assured that I recognize each person's role and appreciate their unique contributions to my journey.

This book took shape and evolved under the skilled editorial mentorship and guidance of Art Joyce and Alex McGilvery. Their respective expertise and understanding helped me immeasurably when I wandered in circles, struggling to get my bearings and move forward towards publication. Anne Champagne's fine copyediting skills enhanced the final manuscript with her adept polishing. I am delighted that Alex from Celticfrog Publishing later welcomed me to hop on his tiny lily pad in the publishing pond.

A heartfelt thank you to Michael Kendrick whose wealth of knowledge, experience and understanding of inclusion is valued globally. By writing the book's foreword, Michael endorsed the merit of our family's quest for ordinary and honoured the warrior spirit required to endure the perilous journey.

Last, but not least, the heart of my book belongs to my immediate family—Neil, Matthew and Kate. Each member represents a rock of unconditional love, unwavering commitment and pursuit of social justice. All gave me free rein to speak my truth, respecting the validity of my perspective. Only when my memory faltered about an incident that directly involved them did Kate or Neil suggest minor edits to ensure accuracy. All members graciously supported my openness about sensitive matters to shed light on challenges that can readily consume struggling families. I am immensely proud of Kate who nonchalantly picked up and donned the mantle of advocate, leading by example with her boundless compassion. Although given the opportunity to review anything I'd written, Matt declined, instead trusting me to be honest, clear and respectful.

My book speaks of nourishment and that's what Neil provided throughout the creative process, from contemplation to publication. Consciously choosing not to influence my writing in any way, he provided both emotional and physical sustenance. Neil nourished me, literally as I sat at the computer, not noticing that daylight waned. During dark winter afternoons, he turned on my light and asked what time I'd like to eat dinner. Then he set off to cook a delicious meal. Without fail, he provided ample countdowns, before announcing that dinner awaited me at the table. Finally, he nourished my soul by using his photographic and design talents to create the *Warrior Angel* book cover.

They say family means everything. I wholeheartedly agree and am eternally grateful for mine.

Introduction

Life is a process of becoming—no exceptions. For those society judges as "different" the process is more challenging. Society erects hurdles that diminish opportunities to achieve a full life. This book offers readers a rare view behind the weighted veil of marginalization, providing an intimate view of one family's journey with disability. Love wears many faces and readers will see them all. Each chapter speaks directly to key themes, real experiences and reflections that span over three decades.

Many people sneak peaks at disability, garnering impressions from quick glances. Innocent children stare and ask "What's wrong with that person?" Parents frequently hush the child or label the person disabled, before hurrying away. Advocates such as me would love to be invited into such conversations, with the goal of educating, not blaming. Ignorance is not bliss and weighs society down, to the detriment of all.

Universally, the recipe for unleashing human potential includes belonging, opportunity and contribution. When devalued societally, access to these core ingredients takes courage, advocacy, and tenacity. My husband, Neil and I pried open the door of belonging for our vulnerable son—and always kept a foot wedged there. Our quest was for treasures embedded in ordinary life. Extracting beauty from "ordinary" takes time and grit, like creating a pearl within an oyster.

Layers of human complexity impact all lives, some more than others. This book's personal stories address all aspects of our family's daring expedition, without sugar-coating. Readers will be exposed to the panoramic landscape, through an unfiltered lens. Diverse experiences and emotions have been laid bare, reflecting the unpredictable rollercoaster ride of good, bad and otherwise.

While each story is uniquely ours, the inherent themes are commonplace for devalued populations. Anyone who thinks

1

marginalized citizens are unaware of their devalued status has not walked the rocky path with a loved one. Every success story of inclusion has been hard earned, with risks of losing grip never far away.

The boundaries of marginalization are fluid and can affect anyone, at any time—life's luck of the draw. Intellectually we know that youth, beauty, fame and fortune can turn on a dime, yet societally we negate it. Accidents of birth, traumatic injury, gender identity, and diminished capacity—it matters not. Looking beyond labels, one gains insights about hurdles to an ordinary life, when someone is defined as "different."

In our family's case the label is disability. People wear blinders when looking at those of us impacted directly or indirectly by disability, even when well intentioned. Innocent questions such as "What does he have?" are seeking simple answers to complex issues. What our son Matthew has is a *life*, significantly impacted, but not defined by disability.

Our eldest is a kind, sensitive and vulnerable citizen. His primary, but not sole diagnosis, is Williams Syndrome. This obscure, multifaceted developmental disability is caused by a random genetic anomaly. The syndrome casts a wide shadow, with physical, intellectual and emotional health implications. Each person has many, but not all the diagnostic traits, impacting their whole being, to varying degrees.

Unfortunately, our son lives in a society that values everything that disability is not—and he knows it. At times Matt rages against the world that coats him in humiliation and taunts him for not being good enough. He sees what others his age have and he wants so badly to break through the glass ceiling to ordinary.

Our family's trek is about balancing on a razor's edge at Matthew's side. We do our best to nurture and support, while holding him to account for becoming the best man he can be. Like an artist's abstract painting, brush strokes blend layers of darkness, brilliance and clarity. As the artwork progresses, nuances surface, while tints and texture draw us further into Matt's unique being.

Well embedded in adulthood, our family does not treat Matt as a *man-child*. His sister, Kate, is particularly good at identifying any slippage. Admittedly all of us sometimes give leeway, due to Matt's cognitive challenges, while striving to avoid "special treatment." Neil and I understand natural family temptations to wrap a vulnerable person in cotton wool. However, everyone wants and deserves more in life. In reality, our eldest is safest by his being armed with personal skills and attributes to walk among us, with ready access to personalized resources that help him navigate life.

For many years, people said to me: "Matthew will always need you. So you'd never consider moving away, right?" Their long-term perspective didn't match mine. Yes, he needs me in his life and I need him, for as long as we're both on this earth. However, he does not need my physical presence hovering over him. Neil and I now live a 10-hour drive away from Matt. Our son is secure in the knowledge that we're available to listen, understand, console and clarify at any time. The metaphoric mantle of warrior angel gathers no dust hanging in our family's closet.

I'm definitely not saying that we are angels—far from it. However, the protective traits of a warrior angel lie within all of us. Whether a dormant spirit or not, every citizen has a personal trigger that can rally their courage to raise a voice and stand up for an underdog. Nurturing a warrior angel spirit increases the odds of a vulnerable person thriving—not just surviving—in life.

Angels are typically depicted as being loving, pure, selfless and all forgiving. In short—perfect, therefore not human. In real life, traits of angelic radiance and light are counterbalanced by the fierce warrior component, fuelled by relentless determination to battle injustice. Inclusion is our battle cry.

Being ever vigilant is exceedingly taxing on relationships, time and patience. Admittedly, I'm not always fully engaged, proactive or sensitive. I'm simply doing my best, at that moment in time. It still doesn't stop me from berating myself.

Sharing my human transgressions with a kindred spirit on their own unique quest is invaluable for regaining perspective. The power of nurturing such an advocacy network cannot be overstated—another key theme in the book. Alone, yet not alone.

Disability challenges have far-reaching impacts on our son's life. However, what's equally challenging is society's overarching discomfort with difference. Going it alone would be an arduous journey Matt could not sustain long term. However, with the love, support and guidance of family and a support network, Matt's life can reflect the elements of ordinary. That achievement, as tenuous as it may be at times, allows all family members freedom to live their own unique lives in different communities.

Like everyone, Matt needs to fulfill valued social roles as a contributing member of society, rather than someone people dismiss or merely tolerate. At times, he's been well embedded, contributing to the kaleidoscope of community. The fragility of the image can and does change, sometimes initiated by a seemingly small twist of life. Suddenly a new image appears.

For those of us privileged in society, by virtue of race, gender, intellect or wealth, focusing on marginalization might seem like mere political correctness. Actually, it's about humanity and respect. Like trees, we need to bend to the winds of life, standing together and entwining our roots for strength, rather than sacrificing those viewed as less desirable. I invite you to consider our family's struggles and triumphs, while appreciating the tenacious spirit of warrior angel families around the globe. Adoration, pity and ignorance are unwelcome—detrimental forces that impede our progress.

Since the dawn of time, love, determination and ingenuity have made people stronger than they thought possible. We are no exception. The secret to success is perseverance and effort. Our family is intimately familiar with disability and its societal ramifications. Lessons have been deeply painful, heart-warming, insightful and invaluable. Our rocky, challenging path holds the promise of something better. The human condition is such that there is no worry-free lifetime guarantee.

In our family, every member remains true to their beliefs and never compromises on core values, Matt included. We are all stronger for the tests and the lessons have transformed us at some level. Best of all, the values of diversity and inclusion have been passed on to the next generation, our beautiful grandchildren.

The mantle of warrior angel, woven with threads of unconditional love, was unexpectedly placed on my shoulders. Life rarely rolls out like a red carpet, particularly for someone society devalues as "different." I learned to embrace advocacy, rather than accepting the readily offered scraps of less than ordinary for our son.

Candid accounts split open our family's protective outer shell, exposing our soft underbelly. Navigating through societal barbed wire fences and system hurdles, we learned that advocacy has the power to unlock possibilities for a fulfilling life.

The door to our house is wide open—with no tidying up. The stories aren't sequential, so feel free to let your heart lead. What binds chapters together is the focus on challenging low societal expectations and seeking equity of opportunity. The dangling golden ring is the possibility of an ordinary life, as "one of us." The blanket of *belonging* can enwrap all. It's time to welcome people in from the cold.

Section 1. Growing Up

Grasping Realities

Chapter 1: Puzzle Pieces

Developmental milestones were delayed. Uneasiness lingered in the air, despite the public health nurse's reassurance.

"Nothing to worry about. All babies progress at different rates, on a wide spectrum. Matthew's muscle development is simply starting out lower on the scale." Smiling, she recorded his progress and handed back his developmental report card.

Subsequent check-ups didn't boost our son's percentile ratings. Neil and I were routinely told that a developmental spike could soon be a reality. It was Matthew's beloved uncle who first articulated a pea-sized concern that was taking hold in our hearts.

Within moments of arriving for a visit, twinkly-eyed John picked up our precious firstborn. "Come on there, little man, hold your head up for your good ol' Uncle John." His twinkle vanished and his words became crusted in concern. "Head's still pretty wobbly. I hope you're getting him checked out. Something doesn't seem *right*."

Neil's sister, Isabel, shot a thunderbolt of rebuke in her husband's direction. "John! Who made you a doctor? Every kid's unique—ours are proof of that!" She dismissively waved a hand in his direction. "Don't pay any attention to his nonsense."

They left shortly after. Gentle, well-intentioned John knew he was in the doghouse with Isabel. We chuckled about his predicament, but shared his unease. Thankfully our trusted family doctor had referred us to a seasoned paediatrician. The appointment was four days away.

The doctor's laidback approach implied that as new parents, we were unduly concerned about our son's delays. Matthew's percentile ratings dipped further down the scale, not up. Professionals continued to reiterate that reaching new milestones was likely just *around the bend.* Meanwhile, we relished the development of his new skills.

Matthew's rolling prowess astonished us. He couldn't yet hold his body up to crawl, but rolled like a race car driver, getting places faster than we could walk. Once he learned how to pull himself upright Matthew clung to walls or our hands. But standing unsupported and maintaining balance proved too challenging. Rather than falling over, he plopped himself on the floor, gave his infectious grin and waited patiently until we helped. Developmental strides continued to elude us, month after month.

At 18 months, the paediatrician referred us to Edmonton's Glenrose Rehabilitation Hospital. The appointment was with a physiatrist, a specialist in the diagnosis of physical challenges. Ten agonizing weeks passed before we sat in the examining room.

The physiatrist was intensely focused while thoroughly examining Matthew. He lifted arms, legs, checked foot structure and limb dexterity. Silently like mice, we peered from the corner. Occasionally Dr. Watt paused in contemplation, rubbing his chin with his right hand. Suddenly he grasped Matthew's feet and inserted both heels in their respective ears—toes pointing outward. Our eyes popped, while Matthew grinned.

Before turning to us, Dr. Watt assured Matthew was returned to a balanced sitting position. "Matthew's incredible flexibility tells me a lot."

That got Neil's attention. "His flexibility seems to impress everyone. But aren't all toddlers pretty flexible?"

Dr. Watt smiled kindly and placed Matthew's heels in his ears again, saying "Certainly not to *this* extent." Matthew didn't waver.

I spoke up. "Doctor, we practice walking with Matthew every day. He takes steps fine until we let go of his hands." I couldn't hide the trepidation in my voice. "Will…will he ever be able to walk independently?"

"Yes, I am confident that your son can learn to walk."

"Oh, thank God! But why is it taking so long?"

"Let me explain. The key is in the approach. Matthew has extremely lax muscles and loose joints. With good intentions, you've been letting go after helping him take some steps. However, he needs consistent physical assistance to gain more strength and stability. He'll let you know when it's time to let go. With this new approach, Matthew should be walking independently within a couple of months."

I squeezed Neil's hand, then scooped up Matthew from the examining table. I kissed and hugged him with relief, trying to suppress guilt over our misguided approach. The doctor's explanation made so much sense. Rather than nurturing walking skills, we'd been inadvertently abandoning our teetery toddler.

"Okay sweetheart, we're going to do things differently." Matthew beamed, nestling in my arms. That impish grin soothed my strained heart—no apology or guilt necessary.

Dr. Watt continued. "Besides the developmental delays, there are facial 'pixie-like' features that concern me. It warrants investigation of a rare condition called Williams Syndrome, which has among other things, numerous physical implications. But let's not get ahead of ourselves. The only way to diagnose is with a cardiac catheterization. I'll refer you to a paediatric heart surgeon." The powerful blow hadn't fully registered, just the initial sting.

Once in the hallway, I expelled the toxic message. "Hon, what pixie-like facial features? Matthew doesn't look like a pixie at all. Feels like a far-fetched description."

"One day at a time. Sounds like Dr. Watt wants to explore anomalies that can elude us as new parents. Loved his confidence that Matthew can learn to walk."

"Yet...he's raised more than our hopes. I desperately want to understand Matthew's challenges, but raising the prospect of a rare syndrome? Makes me shudder."

Neil opened his protective embrace. With me cradled under one wing, and Matthew the other, he said, "It scares me too. But Dr. Watt has started us on a promising path to get some answers. Learning that Matthew has lax muscles *and* loose joints is enlightening. We're the key to helping him develop muscle tone and strength. So let's get started." On that note he put Matthew down. Walking the long hallway, we each held a little hand firmly in ours.

Once at home, I turned on the dining room light, closely examining a cherished portrait that Neil took. It was of my grandmother struggling to hold a wiggling and exuberant Matthew, at about 12 months old. I was haunted by the notable depressions above his cheekbones. Whenever I mentioned my unease, Neil blamed poor lighting and an awkward camera angle. An inner voice was telling me something different. Dr. Watt's concerns had a stranglehold on my heart.

At 23 months, Matthew started walking independently. Sighs of relief quickly turned to gasps, as our son took full advantage of this new independence, stretching for everything within his new sightline. Our delayed parental introduction to typical childhood development had begun.

The long-awaited manila envelope arrived from the cardiology department. Comprehensive information included the date, preparation and details about the hospital stay. Those were the days when parents weren't accommodated to stay overnight. We wouldn't be deterred. Kinks in our necks and sore backs from the uncomfortable bedside chair were small prices to pay.

In consultation with the paediatric cardiologist, we authorized the insertion of a catheter through an artery in Matthew's groin and up into his heart. It was the least intrusive procedure for investigating if Matthew had this rare syndrome. The procedure would determine if there was an aortic stenosis, a narrowing of the aortic artery. There was a small risk that the catheter insertion could induce arterial collapse and pose future issues—a necessary gamble.

We didn't leave Matthew's side. Neil printed our son's name at the bottom of his first piece of artwork, a pre-operative masterpiece. We framed the bright swipes of colourful paint with an equally vibrant yellow frame, still a treasure. Sunny days ahead—perhaps.

The anaesthesiologist explained the procedure. He stressed that we could not be present when he was sedating our son. Neil broached the subject gently.

"If we aren't close by, our son will likely become incredibly insecure and upset, invoking skyrocketing anxiety." The doctor's vacant eyes looked through us. Neil clarified. "Having uncontrolled adrenaline coursing through Matthew's body would neutralize what might otherwise be a normal dosage. Our reassuring presence while you administer the sedation could help a lot." Neil's eyes were on high beam.

The anaesthesiologist cleared his throat and dismissively replied, "Don't worry. I know my job. I'll give him a little extra medication if needed, although I expect it'll be fine. We should go now."

Neil and I exchanged knowing glances. We reassured Matthew and walked alongside the gurney until we reached the doors to the restricted operating area. "Sweetie, you're going with the doctor for a few minutes. After a little nap he'll bring you straight back to us. We'll be waiting."

We kissed our son's forehead before he was whisked away. Within 10 minutes, the anaesthesiologist sheepishly sought us out.

"Matthew's not succumbing to the anaesthetic and is inconsolable. There's no proceeding unless he calms and I'm not comfortable increasing the dosage further. Although highly irregular, I'm inviting you in to help reduce his anxiety. That's our only hope if I'm to prep him for the surgery."

With his dad leaning into Matthew's ear on one side of the operating table and me bent over on the other, we gently and repeatedly sang his favourite song, "Baby Beluga" by Raffi. His body visibly relaxed with each rendition. After singing it about 20 times our raw, cracking voices ached for mercy. We croaked and squeaked out a few more verses until our babe was fully sedated. The anaesthesiologist's perfunctory nod sent us back to the waiting room.

After a prolonged period of hall pacing and clock watching, the surgeon appeared. "The procedure went well and revealed that your son's aortic vessel is fine. Personally, I am not convinced that a stenosis should be the definitive marker for this syndrome. Your son may still be diagnosed with Williams Syndrome one day, once more markers are identified."

Unable to ignore the cardiologist's caveat, I craved more knowledge. The internet wasn't yet a reality so finding information on this rare condition was challenging. Somewhere I stumbled upon a British magazine article, titled "My Wild Child." The picture was of a smiling young teenager. The mother described her son as having a propensity for unpredictable emotional flares, while kind and gentle at heart. The boy was identified as having Williams Syndrome.

Our paediatrician dismissed the article. "Remember, Matthew has no diagnosis and the article doesn't offer any insights into his challenges. Torturing yourself like this doesn't help. I suggest you throw it away and move on." Neil supported that stance.

Still, I felt a bond with this mother from across the Atlantic. Like me, she long-awaited answers about her sweet son, prone to exaggerated emotional sensitivity. The lack of answers continued to haunt and challenge Neil and me as a couple.

Year after year, our calendar was riddled with medical appointments, many at the University of Alberta Hospital. Genetic testing, kidney functioning and blood work were all routine appointments. Speech therapy and psychological advice on behaviour management were thrown in for good measure. Gross and fine motor coordination challenges impacted all aspects of childhood development and self-care skills. Less obvious impacts included compromised control of muscles, both large and small, including the sphincter and mouth.

Slushy speech, loose lips and an abundant flow of saliva continued well past toddlerhood. As a preschooler, absorbent wristbands that matched shirt colours discreetly served to wipe his slightly parted lips. Much like a soother that gets retired, the drool cuff was gone before grade one. Parental and teacher prompts cued Matthew when his brain was busy concentrating elsewhere. Far better than wearing a drool cuff.

Blood work was routine and Matthew's reaction routinely dreaded. He was terrified of needles from a very young age. During one hospital appointment with our four-year-old, we were casually handed yet another requisition form. After assurances that the blood work was essential, we braced ourselves—literally. It took fine-tuned teamwork from Neil and me to pin our preschooler long enough for the nurse to draw the vial of blood.

Holding our youngster on his lap, Neil tried to soothe him. "I've got you, Matthew. Promise we'll be out of here lickety-split. Then straight home for a nap. Hope you'll let me join you."

Cradling Matthew both verbally and physically, Neil strategically wrapped his arms and legs over Matthew's, leaving no smidgen of wiggle room. This swaddling of limbs would reduce the risk of injury from the inevitable flailing. I struggled to straighten our son's arm, as Matthew caught sight of the needle. Meanwhile, the nurse made numerous attempts to poke the miniature moving target. Sweat and sadness oozed from parental pores. Our young child could not comprehend why we were holding him captive, especially when he was so scared.

Blood-curdling screams echoed throughout the open-concept hospital, as security rushed in to investigate. What they saw didn't match their imagination. We weren't wrestling a gorilla, but a pint-size four-year-old. We looked like cruel parents and felt like it too.

Filling a requisition for a blood test seemed so simple to others. We knew better.

Despite extensive testing, answers remained elusive. Occasionally we learned something new. One test revealed that the cardiac catheterization procedure as a toddler did result in a collapsed artery. The doctor shared that the impeded circulation further complicated bodily issues, even at a tender age. As if delivered by a tuning fork, the message reverberated to my core. My throat constricted and ached for release as I fastened the last button on our six-year-old's coat. Matthew put his little hand on my arm. His gentle eyes looked lovingly into mine.

"Mummy, I don't want to see that doctor again. He made you sad."

"Oh sweetie, he's a nice man. It's just the information that's sad. But now we know why your right leg and foot get so cold."

"But knowing is good, right? Heard him say blood doesn't go down my leg very good. But that's okay. It doesn't hurt—just gets freezing cold. Maybe I can walk faster to stay warm and wear an extra sock. Would that make you feel better?"

I kissed his head and tousled his hair. "You, my love, make me feel better. Who's turn to push the elevator button?"

In grade one, Matthew's challenges with gross and fine motor coordination difficulties were notable. His exuberance as well as sensitivity to emotions and noises were hard to contain, regardless of the setting. Burnt toast at home triggered the smoke detector and the noise seemed to pierce Matthew's eardrums. At school, he tentatively rushed past fire alarms for weeks after fire drills. Every sight and sound equally vied for his attention. Leaves blowing by the window in a gusty wind captured his attention, as much as the teacher's voice.

In the second grade, the school engaged a behavioural consultant to assess Matthew's difficulty staying focused. Neil and I independently completed a behavioural questionnaire, as did his teacher. The consultant reviewed our feedback and observed Matthew in the classroom. He was amenable to discussing his report findings in person.

During our meeting, the consultant cited an observation that reflected everyday occurrences at home. "Mrs. Dunnigan, I showed Matthew a flash card of a log, in a word association exercise. Typically, children say wood. Matthew used the term lumber and then launched into the recent opening of the store, Beaver Lumber, and what great sales they had. It was extremely difficult to get him back on task."

"That sounds like our boy all right."

The consultant recommended following up with our paediatrician. In turn, he once again referred us to the Glenrose. Hospital assessments were becoming more and more commonplace. Time off work, parking issues and long waits were equally routine.

Such appointments often ended with comments such as, "Hmmm, Matthew is outgoing and hard to definitively diagnose. He's at once precocious and socially engaging, yet presents with baffling physical and emotional challenges. We'll continue to keep an eye on him."

Words poured from their mouths like a pitcher of water and we were the receiving vessel. Too much water and too small a glass left our family drowning, with no shut-off valve. Four years younger than Matthew, his sweet sister Kate joined us in treading water, while awaiting her turn to swim.

I clung to the glass half full approach, which is my nature. Maybe, just maybe this next Glenrose appointment would help, like the earlier one with the physiatrist. This time we'd see a developmental paediatrician.

Dr. Goulden was relaxed, thorough, understanding and forthright. "Based on all of the evidence, I'm confident that Matthew has Attention Deficit Hyperactivity Disorder (ADHD). I'll give you a prescription for Ritalin, which should make it easier for him to tune out extraneous distractions and focus. I'll start with a low dosage and monitor closely."

I gasped. "Ritalin? At seven years old? I'm struggling to comprehend. Isn't there another option?" I looked pleadingly at the doctor and Neil.

"Mrs. Dunnigan, I understand your hesitancy and am not recommending this lightly. From what I've read and observed, it is difficult for Matthew to keep up, for reasons beyond his control. Ritalin is a resource, not a panacea, but it should help."

"If you think it's the best way to go, it's worth a try," Neil said. "God knows nothing else has helped." I winced.

Perceptive, Dr. Goulden rested his chin on his hands and leaned in to smooth the wrinkles of marital discord. "It might help to think of it this way. If you were driving in icy winter conditions with bald summer tires, you'd likely be hard pressed to keep the car on the road. Probably white knuckling it too. Right?"

No words were needed. We nodded, wondering where this intriguing analogy was going.

"Okay, now picture having good winter tires on the same road. You'd relax somewhat and be better able to focus on what's happening up ahead. Think of Ritalin as Matthew's winter tires." With that he laid his pen beside the prescription pad and waited.

Dr. Goulden's analogy made perfect sense. We left with the prescription. The next morning, Matthew agreeably took the small pill with his breakfast. We didn't say why and he didn't ask any questions. At the doctor's suggestion, we didn't mention it to the school either. Didn't want to bias anyone.

All day long, I wondered if the medication was helping or if it was too early to tell. Finally, my workday ended and I picked up the kids from school and daycare.

I tried to sound casual. "So Matthew, how was school today?"

"It was good. Kinda funny too."

"Funny how?"

"My brain didn't want to run all around the room today. That's never happened before."

"Well that's impressive. Maybe you'll start getting more days like that. Was it easier to listen to the teacher?"

"Think so. Mr. Hanson smiled lots and gave me a pat on the back when I left." The Ritalin helped Matthew's focus at both home and school for the next few years.

Always seeking typical ways of enhancing our son's gross motor skills, during elementary school we enrolled him in soccer, swimming and karate. In these environments, effort and perseverance were all that mattered. Swimming was the most natural sport for Matthew. Every Saturday morning he and Kate had a class at the local YMCA.

Eight years old, Matthew was ready to test for his next rank. It required treading water for three full minutes. Everybody, including the instructor, recognized this as a significant challenge for Matthew. We'd try it anyway. That morning our whole family attended his class.

En route, Matthew announced, "Bet I can do it. I become an 'Odder' when I pass." Neil chuckled. "Actually, it's called an otter. It's a special creature that lives on the land, but loves to swim underwater to catch fish. He's long and slim just like you, so that's a good badge to earn." Forever the teacher.

With all but the final test component completed, the caring instructor looked at Matthew and then the clock. "Okay, you ready? Jump in when I tell you. The second hand on the clock will need to go around three full times before you're done. I believe in you, no matter what. Just do your best. Now ready, set, go...."

Time seemed to pause between seconds, but eventually one minute passed, then two. Matthew's legs slowed and his head repeatedly dipped below the surface as the three-minute mark neared. Collectively holding our breath, the final few seconds elapsed. Clapping erupted and the instructor waved him to the side of the pool. Buoyed by his accomplishment, Matthew got a second wind, smiled, swallowed more water and kept going.

Neil cupped his hands around his mouth and shouted. "Ahoy Mr. Otter, stop bobbing for fish now and we'll take you for a pancake breakfast."

Shaking his head, Matthew sputtered, "Wanna do more..." Then his blond head disappeared underwater. Sculling his arms and hands, Matthew resurfaced and stared directly at the clock. Our cheers grew with each passing minute. Tenacity and success spurred him on. Amazingly he treaded water for 12 minutes—four times the goal!

Exiting the pool on spaghetti legs, our proud athlete turned to his dad. "Think I earned a giant pancake *and* chocolate milk."

"No problem. Maybe I'll have one too. Just watching you tired me out." With that, Neil tossed a towel over Matthew's shoulders and escorted our shaky boy to the changeroom. While waiting, Kate and I pondered our celebratory brunch options.

Juggling the demands of a career, home life, family business and specialists' appointments had me stretched taut, like a balloon about to burst. One memorable day at work I got another cheery phone call from the University of Alberta.

"Mrs. Dunnigan, I'm calling from the genetics clinic. We haven't seen Matthew for a couple of years so want to schedule a check-up. When's a good time to come in?"

Work was a pressure cooker of projects and meetings. There was no good time. Putting my head in my hands and staring at my full calendar, I pushed back.

"Forgive me, but probably much like your job, I have too many competing priorities and not enough time. For years we've sought insights into Matthew's challenges, with limited success. Every professional finds his symptoms puzzling but lacks answers." I paused for air. "Sorry that my frustration is showing. But you'll need to convince me why I should make this appointment." Silence invited her response.

"I understand your frustration. Unfortunately, sometimes getting a diagnosis takes quite a while. As a child ages, symptoms often become clearer. In the end, perseverance is what points us to a diagnosis. Now that Matthew is nine, we think it's worth another assessment. Does that help?"

"Actually, it does. Sorry if I snapped. Let's see how we can make my schedule mesh with yours. If possible, my husband will come too."

When we arrived for the genetics appointment, a bubbly young nurse promptly appeared and led us to the examining room.

"Matthew, I'll take some quick measurements for the doctor. Let's start with your height and weight."

"Good plan," Matthew replied. "Doctors like to have everything ready when they come in. I know that 'cause I see lots of doctors. Looks like that's a new kind of blood pressure cuff. Wonder if he'll use it…or maybe you?"

Her shrugged shoulders, wink and sparkling blue eyes left him guessing. He grinned in return. After measuring Matthew's height, the nurse turned to me.

"Mrs. Dunnigan, it was me who spoke with you on the phone. I'm glad that you decided to come in. And Matthew, you sure have grown since we saw you last." Then the door opened a crack, allowing a tall, lanky doctor to slide into the room.

Dr. Bamforth was new to us. We immediately liked this man with his distinctly British accent and casual manner. He exemplified empathy, patience and competence. After doing a thorough physical exam, Dr. Bamforth sincerely thanked Matthew for his cooperation and asked if he could talk with us next. That was fine with Matthew, who was eager to inspect more aspects of the intriguing blood pressure cuff.

The geneticist bombarded us with questions that were highly unusual, yet exceedingly relevant to life with Matthew. For the first time ever, we answered a resounding yes to over 90 percent of a doctor's questions. It was surreal.

"Would you say Matthew has any hypersensitivity to noises?"

"Absolutely. He almost needs to be peeled off the ceiling if a smoke detector goes off," Neil said.

"Hmmm, okay. And how would you say he is when encountering strangers—shy, talkative, tentative or overly engaged?"

"Never shy," I answered. "You'd think he knew them forever. In fact, he often initiates conversations with complete strangers." I smiled at Matthew who was off in another world, examining minute details of the blood pressure cuff.

"And would you describe his emotional reactions as subdued, typical or off the scale?"

In tandem we replied, "Off the scale." This incredible line of questioning prompted us to elaborate.

I started. "We witness an explosive rainbow of emotion, spanning fear, happiness, sadness and anger."

20

"We refer to it as the 10-times factor," Neil added. My head bobbed in agreement.

Dr. Bamforth glanced at the nurse who casually slipped out of the room. Within a minute or so she returned, with a brochure in hand. This empathetic man continued asking questions that made my spine tingle. He seemed to know our son intimately.

"Matthew's physical challenges and the descriptions you shared align with the profile of someone with Williams Syndrome. As syndromes refer to a collection of features and symptoms, some are more pronounced than others. Although this particular diagnosis was suspected when he was a toddler, Matthew didn't have a narrowing of the aorta. We now know that's not a definitive marker." The air felt sucked out of the room.

Dr. Bamforth delivered his words softly and deliberately, while not taking his eyes off us. A conclusive diagnostic bomb was ready for detonation. He nodded to the nurse.

Stepping forward with compassion in her eyes, she passed me the brochure, thereby pulling the pin. Amidst the text were pictures of children who could have been Matthew's siblings. The little girl on the front cover almost looked like his twin. The bulleted descriptions of physical, behavioural and emotional challenges were strikingly familiar to us.

Seeing the blend of shock and recognition that descended on our faces, Dr. Bamforth gently continued. "In recent years genetic research of Williams Syndrome revealed the impacts of a micro-deletion, of the elastin gene. The micro-deletion affects all aspects of bodily elasticity. Anything with elasticity is affected, ranging from the heart, to arterial walls, mouth and sphincter muscles. That helps explain the delays and challenges with gross and fine motor skills, slushy speech and so on."

After giving us a few moments to look closely at the brochure's pictures and bullet points, he continued. "You can see by the pictures that there are recognizable physical traits, like there are

21

identifiable traits with Down Syndrome, which is far more prevalent. Lastly, Williams Syndrome includes intellectual impairment, with a wide range of impacts, including highs and lows of comprehension."

The emotional shockwave initially rendered us speechless and dazed. Thoughts swirled, and words struggled to make their way out of our throats. Raw emotions wrestled their way to the surface.

A soft, caring voice wafted into our consciousness. "I know this is hard to process," Dr. Bamforth said. His eyes touched my soul.

Emotions now unleashed, Neil's questions gushed free like a dark, thick oil spill. "What would've caused this? Maybe exposure to the sour gas leak when Susan was pregnant? Could it have been prevented? We have another child—is this hereditary?"

"No blame to place anywhere. This is a random genetic event. It has nothing to do with environmental factors and is not hereditary. Current thinking is that Williams Syndrome randomly occurs in about one in 20,000 births. Of course, as more research is done, we'll learn more and those estimates may change."

I struggled to harness my emotions. Dr. Bamforth handed me a Canadian Williams Syndrome Association business card, with contact information for Alberta's representative. He suggested we reach out to this person who was also a parent. I could only nod my head. If I uttered a word, Matthew would sense my despair.

Leaving the hospital was a blur. I recall holding onto Neil's arm as we navigated the maze of hallways. With Matthew latched onto Neil's other arm; I was protected from our son's line of sight. A heavy stream of silent tears poured down my face. I didn't once try to wipe them away. I bit my lip to repress deep sobs that wailed within. Neil kept Matthew engaged with talk of a treat on the way home. I was alone in my own dark prison of painful thoughts. Yes, I'd wanted answers, but not this....

On that day, key puzzle pieces of disability were connected revealing the mask of Williams Syndrome. While not defining him, the syndrome's prickly tentacles weave throughout all aspects of our son's being. The full range of impacts would unfold for years to come.

At home, I unfurled the brochure and stared at the business card. Gathering courage, I hesitantly called the provincial Williams Syndrome representative. Unsure of my words and dreading the unknown, I dialled. Paralysis gripped me. Two rings later a voice reached out to help.

"Hello, hello…anyone there?"

Fighting the stranglehold on my throat, wispy words broke through.

"Yes, I'm looking for help…."

Chapter 2: Layers Upon Layers

A carefully constructed layer cake is a work of art. Yet when forks delve into its contents, everything changes. Layers meld on the tongue and sometimes a particular taste gets lost in the mix. Once layers are blended, there's no reconfiguring the orderly distinctive strata, the way a geologist is able to dissect the layers of a mountain.

Each person is a well-blended layer cake—messy and unique, with core features. It's something most people take for granted unless someone is discernibly "different." That's when systems and society readily apply labels that pigeonhole and define. This oversimplification is hogwash, but has great mass appeal.

All too often people focus on one facet or another, parts of the whole. The most common questions seek a neat and tidy diagnosis. It's the equivalent of defining a multilayered tiramisu as simply *cake*. A key component for sure, but it's the intermingling with other ingredients that gives each bite its distinct flavour. A bite of Matt's intertwined flavours varies in the same way. His layers give weight and substance to his own being. Unique—just like every human being.

Over the years we've been bombarded with professional assessments that identify elements, while not capturing the elusive whole. Matthew's first diagnostic label of Attention Deficit Hyperactivity Disorder came in grade two. This initial layer later got linked with the Williams Syndrome diagnosis. For many years Ritalin helped with focus and impulsivity. Still, its efficacy dropped with each passing year. The Williams Syndrome diagnosis was received at age nine. It provided an understanding of chromosomal anomalies, common traits, as well as intellectual, physical and emotional challenges—three layers all under one diagnostic umbrella. Learning about the diagnosis' complex traits and impacts provided some key puzzle pieces. Questions aplenty still rattled in our heads about how our son processed daily life. We desperately sought to comprehend his uniqueness beyond a diagnosis.

Behaviour and emotional control challenges are intrinsic to the Williams Syndrome diagnosis. Common issues are well reflected in conversations with other parents and backed up by psychological assessments. One psychologist shared common traits based on clinical research. Themes included: acts young for age, cannot concentrate or pay attention, poorly coordinated or clumsy, confused or seems to be in a fog, talks too much and argues a lot. Matthew exhibited the full range, which contributed to his high score on the hyperactivity scale. "He just needs a firm hand," some well-intentioned family and friends told us. They usually didn't have children. Professionals prescribed behavioural management strategies and medication. God knows we tried it all.

Health and educational systems initiated all assessments for Matthew's first decade of life. In grade five, a colleague recommended a private psychological clinic that our family found useful. It proved invaluable, fostering understanding.

The thorough psychological assessment shed new light on Matthew's complexity. Tests assessed neurological, perceptual, cognitive, linguistic and emotional development. Spiked mountain peaks and low valleys of comprehension created an unusual picture. The assessment reassured and validated our parental appraisal. Matthew is a walking contradiction. Although couched in professional terms, it was deeply reassuring to hear the message echoed from the mouths of experts.

The clinical neuropsychologist's report identified "extreme variability of scores from test to test." Dr. Greene patiently and thoroughly shared results and provided insights. He was the first to discuss the concept of executive functioning and Matt's significant deficits in processing life in typical fashion. It provided another layer of comprehension. Appreciating our son's challenges is one thing. Constantly developing and adapting strategies to accommodate has been far from easy. The air is thin high in the mountain range of executive functioning challenges. Surrounded by jagged peaks, it's rare to find lush valleys to catch one's breath.

We cultivated an early warning detection system and challenged ourselves to find pathways out of seemingly no-win situations. Our guts churned, knowing in all likelihood what would unfold. Matthew's refrain of "Don't worry—everything will be fine," typically added to our concerns. Impulsivity and limited comprehension of risks heaped layers of vulnerability on his back. Our bouts of impatience didn't help either.

In the summer before grade nine, media coverage focused on the risks of Ritalin, shining a light on parental abuse. One could feel the judgement. Early in the new school year we broached the issue with our trusted developmental paediatrician, Dr. Goulden. Per usual, I was the primary spokesperson.

"Rather than increasing Matthew's Ritalin dosage once again, we're wondering about more natural options. Are there any?"

"Definitely. Options abound. What one person swears by might have no clinical testing or evidence of its effectiveness. Conversely, what is well backed by research might not work well for an individual. Only by considering the uniqueness of each person can you find the best match." Looking me in the eye, he waited for the message to absorb.

"And that's why we trust you. We're hoping…well, for something better, I guess."

Dr. Goulden seemed to be reading my mind. Smiling, he leaned across his desk, resting on his elbows and cradling his head in cupped hands. "By the way, being natural does not necessarily mean it's good for you." Mischievously he added, "After all, strychnine is natural."

Smiling, Neil said, "I think you've made your point. So what would you recommend?"

"Well, there is an alternative to Ritalin that's showing good clinical results. My only caution is that in a small percentage of patients it can lead to some heart irregularities. We'd need to monitor closely, specifically for that reason."

We started the new medication on the weekend. After school on Monday I asked Matt how his day was.

"It was pretty good actually. It sounds funny but when I waited at the bus stop this morning, it felt like I had an angel beside me, like my shadow. She stayed there all day too."

The angel shadow helped contain the sloppy hyperactive layer of Matt's cake. A promising sign, but the jubilation was short-lived. Close monitoring quickly detected risky heart irregularities. Other trials didn't prove helpful, so prescription options evaporated. Medication had acted like gelatin, mitigating seepage across all layers of life. Now devoid of such options, we turned our focus to therapeutic practices, such as biofeedback, reiki, massage and chiropractic services. None of these services were eligible for cost sharing, so our pocketbook took a heavy hit.

A second extensive psychological evaluation undertaken in high school closely aligned with findings from the assessment at age 10. Both psychologists stressed how it was easy to overestimate Matt's complex reasoning and problem-solving abilities, thereby placing inappropriate expectations on him.

Limited awareness of social nuances puts Matt at risk, especially when innocent intentions get misinterpreted. I recall an incident at West Edmonton Mall, when he had just turned 11. As a special Spring Break treat our family booked a theme room at the mall's hotel. Both kids enthusiastically chose the Roman Room because of its hot tub. Kate jumped into her bathing suit, while Matt and I hopped on the empty hotel elevator to buy tasty treats at the mall's concession area. The elevator stopped at the hotel lobby, which opened into the upper mall. Three young girls around his age stepped in. It wasn't uncommon for shoppers to hop aboard for the one floor descent to the mall's main floor.

Distancing himself from me, Matthew stepped forward and smiled. "Pretty cool place hey? I'm staying at the hotel. Where do you girls live?"

I stifled a smile, without acknowledging any association. Taken aback, the girls exchanged glances, smiled weakly and looked relieved as the elevator doors opened. They went one way and we went another.

"Still wonder where those girls live. Maybe Vancouver, Toronto or even Halifax. I'd love to visit all those places someday—especially want to visit family in the Maritimes."

"Hopefully you can someday. I don't think those girls travelled far though—probably live here in Edmonton, like us. Sometimes shoppers at this end of the mall take the hotel elevator down. It's closer than walking to the escalator and backtracking."

About 10 minutes later, Matthew was still admiring the snack selection while I finished paying at the kiosk. My spine tingled, so I turned around. The girls stood at the food court entrance, with a mall security guard. They pointed at my son and started walking in our direction.

As they got closer, I joined Matthew's side. Now within earshot, I said "Okay my dear, let's head back to the hotel. Dad and your sister will approve of our purchases."

Stopping dead in their tracks, the security guard mouthed "Sorry" and the girls sheepishly hung their heads. Not mean girls, just too hasty with judgement.

My curious son was not a stalker, but rather an innocent boy, oblivious to personal space and who stood out as being a bit "different." If he'd been buying snacks without me, things may have taken a different turn.

Months later, Matt gave me an unexpected, precious gift. He'd initiated a heart-to-heart talk about something important to him.

Although the subject matter eludes my memory, I do recall him stopping to lovingly address me before leaving the kitchen.

"Thought you should know you're the best mum I've ever had."

"Well, thank you." My face brightened and my body sat a little taller. "In fairness, I am the only mum you've ever had."

"Doesn't matter, Mum—you're still the best."

Holding tightly onto that heartfelt message anchored me through upcoming challenging years. Difficult decisions were made more palatable, affirmed by unconditional love.

The question of applying for legal guardianship and trusteeship loomed as Matt approached adulthood. Our family's commitment has been to nurture independence, where Matt exhibited capacity. Our son never hesitated to reach out for guidance or support with health-related matters, so no need to pursue a guardianship application.

Our concern was and always will be financial. Rather than applying to become his legal trustee, we guided, preferring to try informal approaches over imposing legal control. That path turned into a minefield, yet sometimes you only know by trying.

A head injury at age 20 added more complexity, as reinforced by another neuropsychological assessment. The report spoke to Matt's intellectual impairment, mental health dysfunction and significant limitations with neurocognitive skills. Echoing earlier psychological assessments it addressed the explosive recipe of high stress, anxiety and feeling overwhelmed. When interwoven, their powerful forces can break Matt's floodgates of emotional control.

The layer cake of Matt's life is an ever-changing colourful concoction of intriguing tastes and textures. Full-bodied darkness is balanced by tantalizing light swirls and sprinkled with explosions of creativity, resiliency and innocence. The flavours on his palate change as he forks up each new day and the experiences it brings. What will today's bite of life offer?

School Years

Chapter 3: Welcome to School

Obsessive scrutiny of the classroom door proved futile. There was no vibrant bat for Matthew. A cold granite stone sunk deep into my belly. How could this be, after such careful planning? The boulder's presence felt ominous.

Matthew's early education experience had been shielded, at a small Montessori preschool and kindergarten. Now age six, our vulnerable young son was registered fodder for the public-school system. The plunge into grade one awaited us.

Navigating uncharted waters required a warm, welcoming environment that would recognize and accommodate Matthew's undiagnosed challenges. While cautioning ourselves against letting convenience rule the day, we were eager to explore a prospect close to home and directly beside our daughter's daycare. Maybe too good to be true?

My phone conversation with the principal put me at ease. Exuding warmth and understanding, Mr. Zapach had a particular teacher in mind. We booked an after-school meeting to avoid disruptions.

Neil and I both attended. Being mindful that Matthew was in the room with us, I began. "Our son is a very curious young boy who— as you can see—is full of energy. His milestones were significantly delayed. The combination of lax muscles and loose joints has multiple ramifications, affecting facets of daily life. Examples include not walking until 23 months, difficulty with fine motor skills, some balance issues and so on." I paused for air.

Neil touched my arm and said, "Where Matthew may lag behind in skill development he makes up for in enthusiasm and eagerness to learn."

It was challenging to maintain eye contact with the principal and teacher while simultaneously keeping Mr. Curiosity within my peripheral vision. Engrossed with exploring the office, Matthew looked, touched and inspected a wide array of desk and office accessories. Mr. Zapach didn't seem to mind at all, which helped me relax, at least a bit.

Bending down to his eye level, Ms. Sjoberg introduced herself as the teacher. "So Matthew, how do you feel about going into grade one?"

"Oh I'm ready. I have a new backpack to put homework in. Room for my lunch too. I can trace letters and sing and stuff. And I'm a very good helper."

"Well that sounds great. What do you think, want to see my classroom? I'd like to show you the kinds of work kids do. We can leave your parents to talk more with Mr. Zapach while we're gone." Matthew reached for her hand and bounced down the hall beside her.

Grateful to have private time with Mr. Zapach, we provided clear examples of challenges faced by our son. Topics included Matthew's acute sensitivity to loud noise, anxiety levels, processing challenges, perseverance and impulsivity. Discussion focused on proactive strategies that could discreetly help, without highlighting what separates Matthew as being "different."

Mr. Zapach thanked us for the frank discussion. "Being so well informed will help tailor our approach to support your son's learning and promote inclusion. We can definitely take steps to prepare Matthew for fire-alarm testing, pair him up with a carefully selected classroom buddy and develop other strategies as we get to know him."

An effervescent Matthew returned from the classroom, smitten with Ms. Sjoberg and eager to start school. "I have two questions before we go." He held up two fingers to reinforce his message. "When do I start and…" Standing arrow straight and quivering he added, "Can

I get homework right away?" We all had a spring in our step as we left the school.

All summer, Matthew marked off days on the calendar and dreamed about putting homework in his new backpack. Our pending journey into the educational abyss felt less perilous with a stellar teacher and a progressive principal at the helm.

On the first day of school, Matthew bounded directly to the classroom. His colourful backpack was my beacon when navigating the congested hallways. I caught up with him, staring intently at Ms. Sjoberg's classroom door. He was flabbergasted and his gaping mouth mirrored it well.

The door's creative sign reflected the recent release of the Batman movie. "Welcome Bat to School" hung over fluttering black and yellow construction-paper bats, each bearing a student's name.

"Where's my name, Mum? I don't see it anywhere." Neither did I.

"Matthew wait here by the door, while I go ask the teacher." Anxiety was mounting, for both of us. He was a stranger here, while most kids already seemed to know each other, likely from kindergarten. Had we made a mistake in not enrolling him last year?

My gut churned as I kept one eye on Matthew and the other on the moving target—the besieged Ms. Sjoberg. After not so subtly wedging my way past others to reach her, I heard the explanation.

"I'm glad you nabbed me. Here's the good news. Over the summer another grade one teacher was hired. Fortunately, she has experience teaching children with fine motor difficulties. Ms. Black's classroom is directly across the hall. Sorry to rush, but I have lots of parents still waiting." The enthusiastically delivered news settled that granite stone even firmer in the pit of my stomach.

A confused Matthew reluctantly held my hand and crossed the bustling hallway. It felt like we'd crossed the continental divide.

Bland autumn leaves papering the door reminded me of my own early childhood school years. Matthew automatically offered his hand to greet Ms. Black. Motionless, she looked blankly at him and then at me.

My indignant eyes pierced hers as I suggested Matthew extend his hand further, so Ms. Black could reach it. Only then did she reluctantly offer a limp handshake. Quickly withdrawing her hand, she waved her arm towards the rows of desks. "You can choose any empty desk," then walked away. Distressed, Matthew had gone from bursting with delight to clinging and crying—all within a matter of minutes.

"Just go," was the sole advice Ms. Black offered me, as she walked up and down the rows of desks. After countless reassurances, my distraught son reluctantly released me from his death grasp. Ms. Black ushered me out the door, leaving a scared captive inside.

We had 12 years of public schooling ahead of us. The first 12 minutes were already catastrophic. I foresaw pending disaster unless there was an immediate change. Brave enough or not, I needed to act. My legs found their way to the school office, while my heavy heart remained parked outside the classroom door.

I politely insisted on waiting, requesting two minutes of the busy principal's time. Strong on will, but shaken by the aloofness of Ms. Black, the question kept circling my brain: Who was I to challenge the school's professional assessment? I wrestled with this until the principal's door opened.

Mr. Zapach's warm smile and calm presence cleared the fog from my mind and steadied my nerves. "Come on in. First day of school's always frantic. Hope you approve of our change in teachers. This should help…"

"Excuse me, but I need to interrupt. I appreciate your good intentions. However, with all due respect, I know my son's needs better than anyone. Even educationally, at this juncture I have more expertise than unfamiliar professionals. Ms. Black's unique experience could be a good fit for Matthew's dexterity challenges, but there are so many more factors to consider." I needed to move from generalities to the specific—too much was at stake. "He's currently distraught and crying in that classroom. Matthew made an immediate deep emotional connection with Ms. Sjoberg. I have no doubt that her talents will bring out the best in him. Please trust me on this one and next year I'll try not to be pushy."

Had I gone too far? Daring to look up, I saw Mr. Zapach leaning forward, with chin in hand and listening attentively. With a reassuring smile, he stood up and said, "Leave it with me. I'll see what I can do."

The classroom switch was made at recess and Matthew's precious bat was on the door after lunch. The principal's receptiveness and prompt action laid the foundation for a rewarding year. Matthew loved grade one and loved Ms. Sjoberg even more. Ms. Black's stay at the school was extremely short-lived.

One wintery afternoon Matthew came home looking limp and dejected. "What's the matter?" I asked. "Tough day at school?"

"I'm worried. Ms. Sjoberg was away again—three full days now."

"She's probably got a bad cold, sweetie. Lots of that goin' round."

"Nope, I think she's really, really sick."

"What makes you say that?"

"Well, Mr. Zapach came to our class. He told us other teachers would be taking Ms. Sjoberg's place for awhile. But Mum, how long is a while?"

Ms. Sjoberg was on an extended absence and Matthew missed her deeply. He was thrilled when she finally returned, working afternoons only until fully recovered. He daily inquired about her health and was ever watchful for any signs of a relapse. Even a sneeze was deemed cause for worry.

Until ready to resume her full-time role, substitute teachers covered morning classes. One day after school, Ms. Sjoberg was taken aback when checking children's work from the morning. Surprisingly the math work was already marked, and some answers were incorrectly graded. Appalled at the substitute teacher's sloppy work, she gathered her evidence. Ready to report the matter to Mr. Zapach, she pushed her chair back, and then sensed a presence in the doorway.

Sporting a Cheshire cat grin, Matthew approached. "Finished for the day, Ms. Sjoberg?"

"Matthew, shouldn't you be waiting for your mother?"

"Yah, but I told the after-school staff I'd be here asking you something important. She'll know where to find me."

Ms. Sjoberg queried, "So what's your important question?"

"It's an easy one. Did I do a good job helping you out today?"

Puzzled, she cocked her head. "I'm not sure what you mean. Helping me how, Matthew?"

Opening his arms like a showman, Matthew proudly declared. "By being your assistant during morning recess. That's when I snuck back in the classroom real quick."

"Tell me more."

"Well, I sat tall at your desk and marked all the arithmetic the other teacher left on the desk. I don't want you to work super hard and get sick again. Hope I'm not in trouble...am I?"

"Matthew, you are always a great helper and I appreciate your concern. But marking students' work is a job only for the teachers. And you know that the teacher's desk is off limits to students. Can I count on you to remember that in the future?"

"Yes, Ms. Sjoberg. But I'm curious—did I get most of the answers right?" Alas, math was not his forte.

My footsteps approaching the classroom door served as a diversion. "Looks like you gave good instructions about where you'd be. Here's your mother at the door. Now Matthew, you run along and get your coat." With dancing eyes, she shared why it was my well-intentioned son, not the substitute teacher, who needed to be gently reprimanded.

Although it was hard to leave the radiance of Ms. Sjoberg's classroom, the school had another exceptional teacher in store. For grades two and three, Matthew's learning was nurtured by Mr. Hanson's creativity. Math skills were nurtured as pupils added and multiplied the daily number of diapers needed by Mr. Hanson's growing young family.

In the winter of grade two, the school hired a part-time resource room teacher, Ms. Rowles. Matthew received a few hours of her skillful attention each week. Enthusiasm for teaching exuded from her every pore. She seemed to float down hallways, while acknowledging everyone along the way. Ms. Rowles imaginatively found ways to bring out the best in Matthew, while celebrating effort and perseverance.

Expression through art was her true passion. At the end of the school year, she wrote an encouraging report and invited Matthew to drop by her fledgling art gallery over the summer. Such an invitation could never be ignored. Her vivacious spirit soared in this bright and spacious gallery. Paintings, sculptures and glass cabinets of fragile treasures all vied for attention.

"Ms. Rowles, what's that cool thing way back there?" Matthew asked, pointing to a small shimmering glass globe amidst countless other fragile items, within a deep glass cabinet.

"You have good taste, young man. That's one of my favourites. It's wonderful to touch. Go ahead, reach in and get it." She didn't need to offer twice.

My eyes bulged as I watched my son—with his dexterity issues—weave slender fingers past delicate objects, with surgical precision. He successfully retrieved the cherished object and I resumed breathing.

"Hold it to the light and you'll see how it refracts different colours." Out of the classroom but still the teacher. After meticulous examination, Matthew held it out for Ms. Rowles.

"Go ahead, Matthew. You know where it belongs," she nonchalantly responded. "Hope you come back again over the summer. I'll be getting more things you'd like." No need for a second invitation.

Their bond overflowed from professional to personal. Ms. Rowles masterfully retained professional boundaries, skillfully bringing out the best in Matthew. It was a godsend for us when she assumed regular teaching duties in grade four. There were now two grade four classes, so teachers took turns selecting students. Rather than being chosen last, which was the norm for Matthew, he was Ms. Rowles' first choice. She was the third in a string of gifted teachers who inspired Matthew and celebrated his accomplishments. Under their collective guidance, Matthew and his peers experienced a stimulating educational environment, where every student felt a strong sense of belonging and fond memories were forged. I trusted this school.

Late in grade five, the spectre of junior high loomed on the horizon, scarcely more than a year away. We wanted to draw upon the supportive expertise of school staff to help us plan the next phase of our inclusive education journey.

Mr. Zapach had recently retired, so I approached the new principal, Mrs. Brown. Initially dismissive of my transitional planning idea, she changed her mind early the next week and promptly arranged a meeting.

"Well, Mrs. Dunnigan, upon reflection, you're right. This is indeed a good time to be proactive about Matthew's needs going ahead." There was something vaguely frosty in her tone, something at odds with her perpetual smile.

I pasted a guarded smile on my face. "My husband and I have always appreciated how welcoming and inclusive this school is for Matthew and all students."

She seemed a little uneasy. "Well yes, we do our best. Now, just last Friday the district announced budget adjustments that could affect what we can offer Matthew. We're looking at how to reprioritize our resource allocations."

I resisted the urge to roll my eyes at the bureaucratese. I knew from my own field that when regular words get shooed away in favour of bureaucratic jargon, it's time to take note. Every sinew of my being was suddenly on high alert. Her smile remained, while mine disappeared.

"But don't worry, I think I have a plan that could work for Matthew. There's a program we can get him into. We can enrol him in this special education program—he fits the program perfectly." Her pasted smile didn't even twitch.

A perfectly simple fit, from the system's perspective—quick and easy—but misaligned with my request. I'd requested a plan to foster ongoing inclusion and was being offered segregation, now dressed up as special education. Trying to absorb the principal's recommendation, I reminded myself that junior high represented a huge leap in educational expectations. Was I being unrealistic seeking continued inclusion after grade six?

Before I could collect my thoughts enough to speak, she barrelled on. "Ah, the only slight hiccup is that it means a transfer to a new school for grade six."

"What—not graduate from this elementary school? Matthew has been a pupil since grade one. All his friends are here, and not graduating with them would be devastating. And trust me, making new friends with peers his age is always a challenge, especially in a totally new environment."

Wanting to be open-minded, I reminded myself that this school historically had our best interests at heart. I presumed the prospective school must extend to grade nine, which in Alberta marks the end of junior high. But a disquieting inner voice compelled me to ask. "So he'd graduate from that school at the end of grade nine?"

"Well, no… It's an elementary school like us—kindergarten to grade six." A chasm opened, crumbling the tenuous bridge between her smile and eyes.

Alarm registered in my voice. "You mean he'd only be in that school for a single year? Then he'd have to transfer a second time, when going into grade seven?"

"Well, yes, but of course we'd make that transition as smooth as possible…."

That cold granite stone occupied my belly once more. "Sorry—I'm struggling to understand…. I'll have to talk to Neil about this."

"Of course, of course! It's an excellent elementary school. He'll continue to have access to optional classes like art. The bonus is an adapted curriculum with teachers trained to deal with—ah, 'special needs' kids. If anything, he'll probably get more attention than he does now." She was so focused on sharing facts, that my distress went unregistered.

The next day, Principal Brown jauntily caught me in the hallway after school. Looking like the proud cat that caught the canary, she cheerily chirped that she had proactively contacted the other school about a potential transfer.

"I told the principal that you and your husband are truly loving and cooperative parents. Should I set up a meeting, maybe as early as next week?"

To squelch the raging fire in my gut, I drew in a deep, deep breath. "Thanks for your efforts, but no thank you. We'll continue to explore other options for Matthew's junior high." I turned away and didn't look back. Guess we weren't as cooperative as she'd hoped.

What Mrs. Brown presented as a viable solution was an outdated and ineffective band-aid approach. It had more to do with the education system's ongoing failures than helping kids like Matthew. Worse, it had the power to wreak colossal havoc at an individual level.

The "quick fix, pass the buck" proposal rudely awakened us to the potential for abandonment, when system needs are prioritized over the people they are mandated to serve. Feeling betrayed by the principal late in our elementary-school experience taught us a valuable lesson, yet it was far outweighed by the positive nurturing garnered from the overall elementary-school experience.

Years later, I learned that our original principal, Mr. Zapach, was also the parent of a child with disabilities. Being from an older generation, segregated programming was the only option available to his son at that time. Knowing this helped explain how well Mr. Zapach related to my parental concerns and how he championed inclusion, starting with our son.

Matthew proudly graduated from grade six with his peers, before they headed in various directions for junior high. Matthew was the first child with discernable intellectual challenges to be included in regular classes at this elementary school. Parents and professionals alike watched how Matthew's elementary years unfolded.

His presence educated everyone and his positive experience encouraged others who later walked this rocky path.

I recall one spring day when a mother from our daughter Kate's daycare approached me. The prospect of kindergarten was around the corner for both of our preschoolers. Marigold yearned for her son to have a regular education like Matthew. She was being guided toward a special education program for Brody, who lives with Down Syndrome.

With encouragement, Marigold dared to follow her heart and enrolled Brody in the elementary school. He comfortably claimed a seat next to his good friend, our sweet Kate. Like Matthew, Kate and Brody graduated alongside their peers in grade six. During those years, Marigold and I touched base whenever she had concerns. We commiserated, brainstormed and strategized. Marigold later benefitted from the Alberta Association for Community Living's Family Leadership training series that served our family so well.

Almost 20 years later, serendipity brought Brody face to face with Kate. He immediately recognized her. His enthusiasm was matched by Kate's voice when she called to share the chance encounter. Brody asked Kate for her phone number so "we don't lose contact again." Without hesitation she wrote it down and will await his call.

Our emerging family leadership role was a tiny, undisturbed seed in our hearts prior to Matthew starting school. During those early years, the seed sprouted and grew stronger, with all family members being both nourished and challenged. By the time Matthew left the safe haven of our elementary-school experience, our family was poised to take on the wild world of junior high school. There, our commitment would be fully tested.

Chapter 4: Lessons from the Produce Aisle

To buy or not to buy, that was my dilemma. Grocery shopping stalled halfway up the first aisle, at the bin of limp broccoli. The store demanded an exorbitant price—what my mother had always called *highway robbery*.

A woman interrupted my mindless grumbling, reaching across to snatch the best of the pathetic lot. Disgust bonded us as we exchanged disparaging remarks about wilted vegetables. She carried on shopping while my feet were cemented in limbo.

I admonished myself. "For God's sake Susan, there's no winning here. Grab a bunch, any bunch—time to move on."

Employing body language as a silent protest, I expressed my displeasure to produce department staff. Of course, nobody was in sight. This shopping adventure had already overtaxed my patience. Being accompanied by our impulsive seven-year-old complicated matters. It always took an inordinate amount of time as Matthew scrutinized every aisle—sometimes twice.

Coming out of my daze, I realized that it wasn't just the produce staff who were missing. Like an eagle on the hunt, I scanned the area for our son's glossy yellow raincoat.

Found him—near the front entrance, but heading my way. Noticing the bundle of green in my hand, Matthew waved his arms wildly, then cupped his mouth to send a message. My pronounced scowl didn't penetrate his shield of excitement. His slushy, squeaky message conveyed something about a big surprise.

Using charade techniques, he shook his head repeatedly, crisscrossed his arms and pointed to the broccoli bin. Message received—put the broccoli back. That earned two thumbs up of approval and advanced me to the next round. I really wasn't in a game-playing mood. With exaggerated arm gestures he pointed to the oversized produce doors, then rubbed his hands in anticipation.

Suddenly the swinging doors burst open, releasing a cart of garden-fresh broccoli from the restricted "Employees Only" area.

Matthew waved to the man pushing the cart and then escorted him to my location, bantering en route. After thanking the produce manager for "bringing out the good stuff," Matthew sealed his appreciation with a handshake.

Seizing the moment, I nabbed mounds of firm emerald vegetables and whisked my son away. Within moments a crowd swarmed the produce cart, like bees at a hive. As we left the aisle, I asked Matthew why he'd suddenly disappeared.

"Well Mum, you didn't seem to be doing anything. Staff always go in the 'Employees Only' doors so I went there. Knocked really loud until someone heard me."

"What happened then?"

"It was simple. I asked for the *boss of the vegetables.*"

"And then?"

"Just had to wait a minute. I introduced myself to Rusty—that's his name. Said my mum didn't like to buy old vegetables and I didn't like to eat them either. Asked if there was better broccoli out back. I could see some big boxes of green way in the back. Lots of other fruits and stuff too. It was a cool place. But I knew I wasn't allowed to go inside. Rusty told me to wait with you and he'd try to find some. And he did!"

Usually I was the teacher for my young son. However, on this day our roles were reversed. It was Matthew who demonstrated the wisdom and courage to question, rather than grumble and accept. He went to the source, directly asked for the truth and got it. The price of our groceries paled in comparison to this priceless lesson.

As we kept shopping Matthew approached any customer with wilted broccoli. After his vegetable update, many hurried back hoping to upgrade the quality of their purchase. "I think I helped save a lot of people from eating old broccoli today."

"Yes, you did—us included."

"Wait until Sis hears what I did. You know how much she loves broccoli. It's my favourite too, then brussels sprouts of course. Let's pay and go. I want to show Dad before he goes to work. Hope you picked up enough broccoli for a few days."

"Got what I needed and more. Looks like you picked up extra things that weren't on our list. You know the drill. Run and return them, while I pay." I handed him five of the seven items he'd deposited into the cart.

"Well at least you're keeping a couple of my good choices. Bet I can be back in two minutes."

"Sure hope so. Off you go—and no dilly dallying."

After clearing the checkout, I waited near the exit. My mind wandered and a smile lifted the corners of my mouth. Shopping trips were always unpredictable, so I cherished this sweet win. My thoughts were interrupted by a gentle, playful voice.

"Excuse me." An elderly woman appeared beside me, her diminutive stature countered by her elevated spirit. "Still waiting for your Energizer Bunny? He sure brightens my day every time I hear him telling customers about good deals. Just like a town crier of old. Not a shy bone in his body it seems." She gently patted my shoulder and added, "You've got quite the lad on your hands."

"No doubt about that." Pride nourished my tired body.

Ten minutes later, Matthew returned. I quickly gripped his hand to guide us out the door—no more side trips today. My boy lovingly squeezed my hand and I squeezed back, as if Morse code.

Matthew spotted Rusty restocking bananas. He caught the manager's attention with an exaggerated wave. The manager cheerfully waved back. Funny, that never happens to me....

"Sorry for the long wait, Mum. Got busy talking with people. One customer thanked me and said I was her 'broccoli angel.' It sounded funny, but really I kinda was...."

Chapter 5: Skipping into Hearts

Mr. Enthusiasm was a favourite nickname for Matthew in his younger years. So it was no surprise when he dashed to sign up at his school's Skip-a-thon table. His beloved former grade one teacher coordinated this annual fundraiser. Being well aware of his challenges, Ms. Sjoberg sought clarification.

"Matthew, do you know how to skip yet?"

"Well…not really, but see lots of kids doing it. Bet I could get lots of money from my neighbours."

"I'm sorry but the rules won't let me add your name to the skipping list. To register you'd need to actually skip at the event."

"Oh—maybe I could still ask for donations anyway?"

Ms. Sjoberg gently shook her head.

I had diligently tried teaching our eldest to skip, but his gross motor challenges, coordination and balance issues prevailed. Ineligibility for the fundraiser tugged at Matthew's heart and mind. Dejected, he turned to his strongest school ally, his grade four homeroom teacher, Ms. Rowles. Most people would have focused on helping Matthew accept the decision, but not Era Rowles. Matthew's current lack of skill was quickly reframed as an opportunity.

"Ms. Sjoberg's right; the rules are strict. So I have a suggestion. If you are prepared to work very hard at it, well then…I could teach you!"

It was so like Era to stretch the boundaries of her teaching, consuming her time and not mine. Even though an extracurricular activity proposed specifically for my child, I was not asked to implement her grand plan. Transferring this expectation to the home front would have been a recipe ripe with stress, frustration and failure—for both parent and child. Generously, Era chose a more promising path.

As the Skip-a-thon was only a month away, time was of the essence. During every recess and lunch break, Ms. Rowles and Matthew, with skipping rope in hand, retreated to the farthest corner of the schoolyard. She cheered him on as he practiced, practiced and practiced some more. This teacher's enthusiasm was a match for Matthew's and her belief in him didn't wane. He had no intention of letting Ms. Rowles down or missing the opportunity to raise pledges.

At dinner mid-week, Matthew shared that some curious children meandered over to assess what was going on. "Ms. Rowles didn't hear them, but I did, Mum. 'Look, he can't even skip and he's in grade *four*.' Then they all laughed…hurt my feelings."

"I bet it did." I kissed the top of his forehead. "Always easy for kids—even adults—to laugh at something they don't understand. What you're doing takes a lot of guts. You should be proud of your hard efforts. I sure am."

With encouragement from Ms. Rowles, Matthew learned to ignore the spectators, who kept coming by. They grew in numbers, comments subsided and intrigue mounted. By the end of the week a spokesperson approached Ms. Rowles. "Can we skip with you too?" The impromptu skipping club had its first recruits.

Matthew now had Ms. Rowles and a cadre of skippers giving him tips, offering encouragement and celebrating his progress. As the Skip-a-thon drew closer the skipping club's membership swelled to 23 participants. By the time pledge sheets were distributed, Matthew's name was on the list. He and his skipping compatriots took collective pride in his accomplishment.

With basic skipping skills under his belt and a clipboard of pledge sheets under his arm, Matthew started knocking on doors. Bolstered by the warm reception and generosity of close neighbours, he begged to go farther down the street. He reminded me that the canvassing was for a good cause—fighting heart disease. My reluctance was overcome. Armed with a watch and basic safety precautions, he ran down the street. Within the allotted hour he came home with many more pledges.

The next day Matthew pleaded to canvass the other side of our long street. "Mum, you have to agree that I've behaved responsibly and I'm gettin' lots of pledges." His reasoning and persuasion propelled us into the stretch zone.

Each day he ventured a little farther, revelling in his independence and success. On the last day of canvassing, Matthew was gone longer than I would have liked. His sister and I went looking for him. I spoke to vaguely familiar neighbours from the far end of our street, all of whom had seen him the day before. At times like this, employing a trusted strategy served me best—thinking like Matthew.

We walked around the corner to the next block; a busier street where he shouldn't have ventured and I didn't know anybody. Our boy was nowhere in sight. With Kate in tow, I approached strangers, whether walking their children or working in the yard. When I told them my mission, all knew exactly who I was looking for.

"Oh yes, Matthew. He was at our place a while ago." One young mother said, "He proudly showed he's on his third page of pledges. By now he's probably about halfway up the street. Gotta love his enthusiasm."

"Indeed I do. Let's go find your brother, Kate. It's almost dinnertime."

Kate showcased her natural skipping skills, as we proceeded up the street looking for her brother. She quickly spotted his effervescent jacket up ahead. "I see him, I see him! He's at that blue house with the beautiful flowers. Matthew, Matthew!"

Engrossed with his work, he didn't hear her. Putting my index finger to my pursed lips and winking, Kate understood. With dancing eyes, she took my hand and we quietly approached. Our arrival would be a surprise.

We waited on the sidewalk for Matthew to finish writing up another pledge. We overheard him say, "Thanks, Mrs. Jones, for turning on your porch light. Guess that means it's startin' to get late, so I'd better get home before I get in..."

"Trouble?" finished Mrs. Jones with a cocked eyebrow and barely contained smile. Raising her cane, she pointed toward the sidewalk. "I think you have people waiting for you." Matthew turned to have a look.

"Yup—busted!" Triumphantly, he waved his clipboard and awkwardly skipped towards us. "Dinner ready yet, Mum?"

Our enthusiastic volunteer earned first place for raising the most pledges in his school. Top fundraisers would be acknowledged and prizes awarded at the next school assembly. I ached for Matthew to have his moment in the sun, recognized by students and staff alike. As luck would have it, the timing conflicted with one of his many specialist appointments. Such appointments always trumped everything. As the top fundraiser, Matthew was given the first opportunity to pick from top-tier prizes. The school put it aside for afternoon pickup, after his medical appointment.

When I picked both kids up after school, a vibrating Matthew clutched his chosen treasure. He proudly sat in the back seat and carefully buckled the huge gym bag safely into the seatbelt next to him.

Kate rolled her eyes. "Really, a seat belt? At least I don't need to call shotgun today." She jumped into the front passenger seat before Matthew changed his mind.

"Alright kids, today we celebrate Matthew's big win before heading home. Anyone want Dairy Queen?" I knew it was our son's favourite spot. Both kids hooted with glee. "By the way, we all get to choose our favourite treat." More hooting.

"Mum, because I did the winning, can I have a banana split with extra toppings and don't have to share it?"

"Definitely. You've earned it. Kate, we get to choose our favourite treats too—just not with extra toppings." I glanced in the rear-view mirror and breathed in the contagious pride that radiated from the back seat. Matt lovingly stroked every inch of that bag.

In the parking lot, Matthew unbuckled his prize. He didn't want to risk having it stolen and took the opportunity to revel in his glory with Dairy Queen staff. Kate and I knew that trying to dissuade him was useless. No need to burst his bubble.

Enormous, the black gym bag had a red Jump Rope for Heart logo emblazoned on its face. For over a decade, the bag gathered no dust. It was his go-to bag, regardless of amount, or weight of items stored. Whether bathing trunks and a towel, soccer shoes and team shirt, or a week's worth of clothing for summer camps and vacations, they all fit in.

The sturdy bag dwarfed Matthew's slight build, but never overshadowed his pride from having earned it. Sheer joy was built into its lining. The Skip-a-thon experience reinforced the importance of living in the stretch zone and fostering natural connections. Matthew's active engagement in community life helped embed him as "one of us."

Shortly after the Skip-a-thon we were at the shopping mall. Matthew waved and stopped to chat with someone I didn't know—a common occurrence. I waited within earshot a few steps ahead.

"I'm glad that Sammy's got his freedom back. See ya soon, Debbie—probably on the weekend!"

"How do you know her, Matthew?"

"Debbie? She lives a few houses before Mrs. Jones—you know, on the street where I stopped getting pledges." Reading my mind, he added, "Don't worry, Mum, I haven't gone outside my boundaries since. But next year I do want to go even farther to get more pledges."

"Okay, but what's this about Sammy and why did you say you'll probably see her on the weekend?"

"Sammy's her dog. Poor thing was wearing a neck collar when I got her pledge. He's better so it's off now though."

"And the weekend part?"

"*Really*, Mum? Debbie's been working weekends at the 7-Eleven for months now. You know that's where I like to spend my allowance. Compared to me, you sure don't seem to know anybody in our community."

Given the kernel of truth in his simplistic assessment. I silently thanked unknown neighbourhood guardian angels. Every pair of watchful eyes and ears gave me courage and hope.

Chapter 6: Running the Gauntlet

Neil called it "running the gauntlet." That dreaded daily ordeal of walking past the canopy of young teens lining the junior high school entrance. Nobody raised their head to say "Hi," nor did our son lift his head from his chest. Neil kept vigil from the car to ensure safe passage.

With elementary school behind us, Matthew, now called Matt, entered junior high school for grades seven to nine. Although most of his elementary peers transitioned to the closest junior high school, we chose a smaller school farther away. One influencing factor was the availability of a designated classroom, with a modified curriculum—the dreaded special education classroom. It was our backup plan, something we hoped to avoid.

We preferred to live in the stretch zone, maximizing learning potential. Still, we wondered if Matt's inclusion in the regular classroom might prove too big a leap. As it turned out, between our registration and the first day of school, the designated program was relocated to another school. Goodbye backup plan. Once again Matt blazed the trail as the only child in the school with a discernible developmental disability.

Like his peers, Matt knew junior high was a big step in growing up. Impressive-looking textbooks, multiple teachers and choices in classes were all part of the initial allure. In his first week, Matt proudly showed me his math textbook. The curriculum launched into advanced work beyond Matt's comprehension.

"You know Matt, this math looks pretty tough. Think maybe I should talk to the teacher?"

Perched on the kitchen counter, Matt clutched the book like a gold nugget. "No, Mum! I'm sure I'll be able to do it. I like this book— please don't talk with her." Reinforcing his point, Matt noted that the book's initial review chapter had familiar-looking math problems from grade six. Not making any headway, I tried a different approach.

"Well let's see what math you do remember. Can you add seven plus eight and tell me the answer?"

Laying down the book, he became very pensive and focused on counting his digits, over and over again. Retaining numbers in his head that exceeded available fingers took all of his concentration, yet an answer eluded him. After several attempts he exhaled deeply.

Matt's hands descended from his face to his lap and a calmness washed over him. He sat taller and confidently looked me in the eye. "Ya know, I'm not really quite sure of the answer…but what an *excellent* question." After a week the coveted math book no longer came home. And we spoke of it no more.

Our son's need for additional classroom support quickly surfaced. Within a few weeks, a caring teacher who observed Matt's struggles took me aside. Quietly she suggested that I ask the principal, Mrs. Grey, about accessing specialized funding for extra assistance. The teacher specifically asked not to be identified. The school's September social provided the opportunity. I cornered Mrs. Grey, as she was putting condiments on her hotdog.

My query erased her welcoming smile. "What extra supports? I don't think there's any funding available. Didn't know he had any additional support requirements. No mention on his file."

"You didn't get the report? You should have. When I sat with his grade six teacher in early June, he drafted an overview about struggles and what strategies worked best to support Matt's learning. Once we registered here, the school said they'd mail it to you. I'll call over to see what happened."

The elementary school later assured me that all the information had been mailed. Damn, why didn't I ask for a copy after the teacher typed it up? I set up a meeting with Mrs. Grey to share my recollections from the elementary school's success strategies. Her reception was cool and matter of fact.

"If Matt needs extra help then maybe another school is best for him. We did lose resources last year to support a special needs classroom. Would you like me to look into transfer options?"

"No thanks. We want Matt to have a typical educational experience. I realize that requires creativity and accommodation. But don't we all need some accommodation at times?"

With lips pressed shut, she clasped her hands on the desk. We were done. She was a busy woman, focused on meetings, protocols and running a tight ship. Non-compliant parents were annoying and I already fell into that category.

Standing up to leave, I was snagged by her closing barb. "Mrs. Dunnigan, friends are important in junior high. You shouldn't ever expect him to find that here."

I wanted to react in juvenile fashion, sticking out my tongue and calling her Mrs. McNasty. Biting my tongue, I managed to reclaim adult demeanour before responding.

"Nothing's guaranteed. Minimally I expect all schools to model welcoming environments. Embracing diversity fosters understanding and nurtures citizenship—good for schools, students and society." With that, I walked out of her office, leaving a trail of disdain.

Fortunately, encouraging staff countered Mrs. Grey's bristly approach. I recall one teacher approaching me after a grade seven field trip to the museum.

"Just wanted to say how refreshing it was to have Matt with us. He was fully engaged and asked such insightful questions. That's more than I can say about many classmates who were preoccupied with snickering, side conversations and yawning. Our museum guide was duly impressed and responded with explanations that deepened my understanding too. In turn, I'll try impressing my wife with my new knowledge over dinner," he added with a smile.

The school's library quickly became Matt's sanctuary. The librarian, Mrs. Elbrond, was his greatest supporter. She appreciated Matt's challenges and recognized that he'd benefit from extra individual attention. She unofficially assumed a role in providing extra educational support. We were grateful for every ally, yet still lacked additional classroom help. I simultaneously coveted and feared aide support.

I talked with a close friend who worked in another school system. She loved Matt and understood educational system nuances and strategies that might help us get individualized classroom support.

"Oh Laura, my only concern about Matt having an assigned aide is that he'll be labelled."

"I've got news for you, Susan. Anyone who wants to label him as 'special needs'—or whatever—has already done so. The question is what's more important—getting extra help or avoiding labels? I'd gladly attend a meeting." Seizing this gift, I quickly called Mrs. Grey asking for a meeting to explore options. I did not mention that I was bringing a friend.

Laura's role was to represent my voice if I was overwhelmed, tongue-tied or intimidated. I appreciated her presence, but Mrs. Grey did not. Laura's confidence, knowledge and direct questions clearly irritated the principal. She later told me that my friend was not welcome at any future meetings.

Being welcome or not was a moot point. This experience affirmed what I was just beginning to truly understand. Power is always heavily weighted in the system's favour. Tenacity, determination and advocacy are essential tools for families to help balance the scales. From then on, I always exercised my right to bring an advocate when negotiating with any human service system.

The principal's comments kept replaying in my head. How could meaningful friendships develop with such a negative leader at the school's helm? I sought guidance from the advocacy organization, Alberta Association for Community Living (AACL). The assigned representative strived to build a relationship bridge. Mrs. Grey had no interest in bridge building. She preferred to erect a wall.

Accepting this reality, our best strategy was to target the classroom directly. A receptive teacher allotted time to enhance peer-to-peer understanding. Matt assumed the lead role as presenter. With AACL's guidance we prepared a customized presentation, with bullet points facilitating content and flow. Matt focused on how disability-related challenges impacted school life and how students could support him. For example, lax mouth muscles benefitted from friendly reminders to swallow when focused on a project. That was particularly important in Foods class.

No punches were pulled and the messages were clear. With great pride, Matt gave the presentation solo, without the physical presence of his mother or AACL. Both the teacher and Matt shared that students were receptive, engaged, and asked good questions.

Junior high is a period of life where coolness rules. So hanging out with Matt didn't gain anyone points. That didn't stop Matt's classmate, Kenny. From grade seven on, he became Matt's friend, routinely inviting our son to his house after school and keeping in contact into Matt's early adult years. Kenny even came by with his girlfriend to our backyard farewell party when Matt headed off to college.

Kenny lived a block from the school. He and Matt would throw a football in the field behind the school after classes. Matt, like his Canadian Football League (CFL) namesake, had a good throwing arm. It was a special treat when Kenny's dog ran between the boys, trying to intercept the ball.

Our son loved sharing highlights during dinner. "Boy, that dog drools when he's playing football. Just like when I concentrate hard. You should see him catch the Frisbee too. It's almost impossible to get it away from him—pretty strong dog."

"Sounds like the three of you had a fun time."

"Haven't told you the funniest part yet. Goofy dog came so close to pulling Kenny into a huge puddle. He stopped just inches away. I fell down laughing. Guess that explains streaks on my pants—not lots." Matt swiped dried mud off his pants and onto the floor.

While Kenny was a clear standout, there was another teen, a girl, who took the opposite path, pointedly harassing Matt. Our son referred to Heather as his arch-enemy. She "accidentally" bumped into him in congested hallways, knocking him into his locker or making him drop books. "Mum, I hate it. She calls me names under her breath, making her friends cover their mouths and laugh. Wish she'd just leave me alone."

I spoke to the principal on more than one occasion. She insisted her hands were tied without hard proof and witnesses. She dismissed it as "kids being kids." Heather chose her settings and timing carefully, minimizing risk to herself. One day after school she taunted Matt in a back lane en route to his bus stop. He'd had enough. Taunting escalated and Matt shoved her. If memory serves me, she shoved back, hurled a final insult and walked away with her friend. Matt believed he was simply standing up for himself. The principal saw it differently. Our turn to be called into her office.

"Mr. and Mrs. Dunnigan, Matthew was witnessed accosting another student and we have a zero policy for abuse. Your son will be suspended for three days."

"And Heather?" Neil's voice was cold and his eyes turned steely grey.

"Nothing for her. Matthew instigated by using physical force." The principal straightened papers on her desk.

Neil cleared his throat. "Our son has been consistently provoked by this girl. Abuse takes many forms—not all manifesting in a physical way. Matthew tried using words to stop the ongoing intimidation and harassment. We have too—by coming to you. Our son is not the sole culprit." I cherish such occasions when I get to remain silent. I reached for Neil's hand and squeezed in solidarity.

Both students were warned that further altercations would not be tolerated. They were encouraged to approach parents and administration if emotions erupted again. Nobody was suspended.

Their paths coincidentally crossed again in adulthood. Heather opened up about her personal struggles during junior high and amends were made. Maturity, empathy and understanding lifted their relationship from one of strife to respect and mutual emotional support.

It took time, yet we did obtain funding for a part-time aide support for grade seven afternoon classes. Everyone quickly noticed that Matt became more focused and successful when supported by the gentle and encouraging Mrs. Hill. By mid-November, we had a rhythm that worked.

Since it was helpful to have the part-time aide, we presumed that it would be even more beneficial to have someone full-time. Being a long-term government employee in the human services sector, I knew the importance of researching funding parameters and criteria for decision-making. Playing my cards right, I gathered sufficient evidence and made a case for a full-time aide for grade eight. Matt's current aide expressed an interest in this full-time position. We declared victory too soon. System rules quickly took precedence.

"Mrs. Grey, can you clarify the unsettling rumour that Matt's superb aide is excluded from consideration?"

"Yes, Mrs. Dunnigan. It seems that employee-related matters are quite widely shared. Unfortunately, she lacks the system's prerequisites for a full-time position. I'll be conducting interviews with a school board representative next week."

"In that case, I'd like to join the interview panel given that the position is specifically for my son. How well candidates fit from a curriculum perspective is clearly your area of expertise. However, it's critical to find a good match for Matt, in attitude and approach. I can help identify candidates with that potential." Closing her eyes, Mrs. Grey exhaled a sigh before looking at me.

"Fine, fine. However, we will follow a standard interview process. You will be assigned specific questions." Accommodating her uninvited, unwanted guest, Mrs. Grey carved an inconsequential role, by assigning painfully insipid questions.

Being sidelined, I focused on absorbing everything about each candidate, noting any concerns that struck me. My sole influence was in the post-interview discussion, where I raised relevant points about each candidate. The air was razor sharp, as Mrs. Grey barely tolerated my input and rationale—always eager to move on. The school board representative delicately played the unofficial role of referee.

Every candidate struck me as ill-equipped, especially compared to Matt's current creative and encouraging aide. Palpable frustration built with each interview. Mrs. Grey wanted to hire quickly and I wanted the best match for my son.

After interviews were completed, Mrs. Grey stated that she wanted the final candidate—the person I assessed as being the worst fit. The shock was written across my face. Before I could open my mouth, Mrs. Grey laid down her trump card. "As the principal the decision is mine. We're done here." She pushed back her chair and walked out. A sense of hopelessness filled the void.

Not surprisingly I had a restless sleep. The next morning began with an unexpected phone call from Mrs. Grey. "Hello Mrs. Dunnigan. There's been a change since yesterday's hiring decision. Just to be clear, it's totally out of my hands. A teacher's aide with union seniority has unexpectedly been displaced. Union rules dictate that she automatically be assigned as Matt's aide for grade eight."

60

It had come down to an administrative directive, in compliance with the contractual agreement between the school system and the union. Grade eight was upon us and we were about to be further educated. Neil and I mutually declared grade eight the Year from Hell. The coveted full-time aide was in place, but what a mistake.

The aide, Ms. Willow, not the teacher, now became the primary educator for our son. While remaining physically within the classroom, our son and Ms. Willow were treated as a unique entity—separate, but not equal. It was the antithesis of inclusion. Clamouring to be included and understood, trouble ensued. Matt rebelled against this shadow that never left his side and set him apart as different from his peers. Like an unwanted backpack he did everything he could to shake it. Under the guise of helping, a divider was resurrected, physically separating Matt's desk from his surrounding classmates. Classroom strategies fuelled the flames of a hellish year.

A daily journal was established and sent home, overflowing with negative comments about non-compliance, poor focus and incomplete assignments. Bad days mounted like winter snow. With little accomplished during the day, work was sent home to be magically completed. Wasted days turned into wasted nights. Our family resented the overarching negativity and the aide who shared it. Once again, frustration burgeoned from every source.

A few years later I was invited to speak about inclusive education with University of Alberta students in the Faculty of Education. Grade eight was our ultimate example of how good intentions can backfire when collaboration is lacking. I had every intention of dissecting our disastrous year, until I scanned the audience. Ms. Willow was in their midst, now a student. I couldn't bring myself to embarrass her. I hurriedly reframed my junior high presentation, being careful to minimize the aide's role in how things unfolded.

Approaching me after class Ms. Willow said, "It wasn't fair that Matt had such a tough time in grade eight. I was in a pressure cooker from the teacher and principal to show results and have Matt keep up. With full responsibility placed on my shoulders, I passed pent-up frustration off to you. I hated that stupid daily journal, but the principal insisted upon it."

"If it's any comfort, we hated it more," I replied. My rigid impression of Ms. Willow softened with every breath.

"Mrs. Dunnigan, that stressful year was instrumental in my decision to pursue this teaching degree." She shuffled her feet and hesitated. "You could easily have made me squirm with guilt and embarrassment. Thanks for holding back."

Knowing other students were waiting to talk with me, Ms. Willow flung her backpack over her shoulder and left before I had the chance to thank her. That chance encounter was an unusual gift. It allowed me to release long-held harsh assumptions and judgements of her. Perspective does matter.

After surviving grade eight, Neil and I knew we needed a new approach for grade nine. Exhausted and at a loss for course correction, no plan emerged. A week before school a lightning bolt announcement resulted in a ray of sunshine. It came from an unexpected source—budget cuts.

Mrs. Grey left us a curt phone message. "Due to district budget cuts, the funding for Matt's aide has been reallocated so there will be no assigned aide for grade nine. I'm arranging for you to meet with the assigned grade nine teacher to figure out a game plan."

Matt was assigned to the homeroom of Mrs. Nathanson, another gifted and understanding teacher. And what a game plan she had!

"Teaching is in my blood and I like to challenge all students to bring out the best in themselves and others. That often means a team approach to projects, with me at the helm to keep everyone on course."

This confident, seasoned teacher had a clear plan for actively including Matt. She declined any offers of additional in-class assistance. Instead, Mrs. Elbrond, the librarian with whom Matt had forged a trusting, positive relationship, provided extra support as needed outside of regular class time. Mrs. Nathanson included Matt in all assignments, involved him in small-group work projects with other students, provided clear direction and gave extra encouragement as needed. Classmates gained an appreciation of Matt's unique perspective and creative project contributions, while Matt applied effort and produced higher-quality work. The classroom epitomized the welcoming environment that the entrenched Mrs. Grey didn't grasp.

In early October, it was time for the students' first science test. Mrs. Nathanson drafted a general test, and then proceeded to modify it for Matt. She reviewed both tests to confirm that they addressed the same content. The comparison revealed something striking. It didn't align with her view of inclusion. Without hesitation she rectified the situation.

The next week, a beaming Matt waved his completed science test in the hallway as I approached his open locker. "Look Mum, I passed! Guess that extra studying with Mrs. Elbrond paid off. Does this mean we can stop for ice cream on the way home?"

The afternoon's light cast a shadow on Mrs. Nathanson who stood in her classroom doorway. She gave a friendly wave and motioned me towards her.

"Matt, you finish getting things from your locker. I want to say hello to Mrs. Nathanson. Bet she's proud of your test results."

Mrs. Nathanson shared her revelation. "When I was comparing Matt's modified test questions with the general one, I realized there was only one difference, but it was significant. The scope and content of the tests matched, but my wording of questions and directions was much clearer on Matt's test."

She paused and smiled broadly. Wanting her to continue, I cocked my head and said "So…?"

"So I ripped up the general test and gave the whole class Matt's questions. Every student, regardless of ability, clearly understood each test question. That positioned them well for answering to the best of their ability. Having Matt in my classroom is making me a better teacher in ways that benefit all students." Again, I thought of Mrs. Grey.

Throughout grade nine, Matt was engaged, challenged and felt much better about himself. One day in early June, he came home with surprising news.

"Guess what? I'm getting some time off school later this week. Looks like I can stay up late and sleep in."

"That seems odd. Why's there no school?"

"Well there is for most kids. They have to write grade nine provincial exams."

"Matt, all grade nine students who take regular classes in Alberta are expected to write these exams. Who told you that you don't?"

"Mrs. Grey." Enough said.

"Well I'll get more information when I call her tomorrow."

Mrs. Grey's rationale was that writing these exams would be damaging to Matt's self-esteem. Her words held no ring of truth. The principal didn't want Matt's performance to negatively impact overall school scores. Per usual, I pressed the issue.

"Mrs. Dunnigan, I'm almost positive it's a requirement that a participating student be taking the full curriculum. That excludes Matt by virtue of him not taking grade nine math." Her tone conveyed a "gotcha" moment. Silence hung momentarily in the air, as I processed.

"But math was the only curriculum that Matt didn't complete with his peers. His focus was clearly on developing functional math skills with Mrs. Elbrond instead. Naturally, as the principal you need to comply with school system requirements. However, you mentioned being almost positive. If possible, I'd like Matt to write tests for all subjects where he does follow the provincial curriculum. Can you give me the district contact phone so I can check directly?"

Mrs. Grey reluctantly gave me a contact phone number, stressing that the tests started the next morning. My window of opportunity was slim, with 20 minutes left in the school board's workday. I dialled immediately. I prayed for a potential opening where Matt could slide in, like a single pane of glass. Initial school board personnel were unsure of the protocol. I asked to speak with a senior consultant who would definitely know. She was crystal clear. Matt could write any individual test if he had been taught the curriculum. And yes, she was willing to call the school and confirm.

Matt's homeroom teacher, who understood his writing and style of expression, would be the person who marked the exam. That was the standard process for all students. Knowing this gave me a glimmer of hope and put my mind at ease.

The issue at hand was not about passing or failing, but rising to the occasion. That's where self-esteem comes into play. Matt passed— barely, but that's okay.

"Mum, I'm glad I wrote the tests, even though they were hard. Pretty proud of myself actually." His team of supporters—family, friends and teachers—basked in his glow.

Comforting keepsakes gathered over the years include a heartfelt congratulations card from Mrs. Nathanson. Excerpts include:

Matt, I could always count on you working to the best of your ability, taking responsibility, helping out in any situation, working with Club M.A.D. projects and passing on a smile, a pat on the shoulder, a thumbs up sign or a happy phrase whenever I saw you in the hallways. It has been an honour and a pleasure working with you this year.

Mrs. Nathanson, Mrs. Elbrond and other supportive teachers were the perpetual rainbows that countered administrative stormy weather. Matt experienced times of cold, dark and brightness throughout junior high, culminating with graduation. With a spritely gait, he walked confidently across the stage amidst his classmates. His head wasn't ducked like that of an outlier, but held high as a graduating peer.

A few years later I encountered a young man behind the Safeway deli counter, in the store where Matt worked. This young adult carefully wrapped my order, as if it was something precious.

Handing me the deli package he said, "You're Matt's mum, right?"

"Sure am. How'd you know?"

"I remember him from junior high." He nodded towards Matt who was busy stacking Safeway red grocery baskets. The young man spoke softly as if miles away in thought. "He sure has come a long way."

A welcome flush of warmth enveloped me. "Yes he has." Winking, I added, "As have you…."

Chapter 7: Marathon Man

Two laps down and one to go. The end was in sight—near, yet so far away. Pioneering mainstream educational inclusion had taken a toll. We'd jumped relentless educational hurdles on this track, leaving our legs shaking with fatigue.

Our provincial advocacy organization, the Alberta Association for Community Living, showcased a proud picture of Matt at his junior high graduation. On the surface all looked good. The underlying reality was that we were low on steam and senior high was upon us like a freight train. We were determined to stay the course.

Matt would clearly need individualized accommodation, probably more than in elementary and junior high. As junior high ended, once again there was no transitional support to assist with decision-making. I'm confident that if we expressed an interest in exploring segregation, options would have been laid out like lovely wedding dresses.

It would be up to us to share educational complexities and strategies that fostered success. Apprehension mounted as increased risks and unknown possibilities loomed, like dark clouds on the horizon. The wild frontier of senior high school was intimidating, even before we walked through the doors.

Matt and I made the rounds of local high school open houses near the end of grade nine. We routinely walked away dismayed. These large institutions felt daunting, threatening and cliquish—this one most of all. Within a few minutes, the familiar tap was on my shoulder. "Can we go home now Mum?"

"Yah, think we've seen enough. This was the last one on our list. Time to take a break." Feeling battered by the ordeal, we exited with matching drooped shoulders.

That weekend during dinner with teacher friends, they asked how our search was going. I vented my frustration and they listened attentively. Knowing Matt and caring deeply, they understood our concerns. Allen asked if we'd like to hear his perspective.

"Of course—as if we could stop you." I winked and sipped a glass of wine. "I await your wisdom." And I meant it.

"Here's food for thought. You've undoubtedly noticed that all schools in your search area are gigantic—the norm these days. That could be pretty intimidating for Matt."

"Agreed—carry on."

Neil and I valued our friend's insights. Allen suggested we consider a smaller school he was familiar with, far from our home.

"Seriously? Being on the southside, it's beyond our initial search area, so not remotely on our radar." That information didn't deter Allen.

"Maybe broaden your scope," he said. "Would mean more travel time and likely at least one bus transfer. But it's got the distinct advantage of being *so* much smaller than enormous schools where you almost need a map to find your way around. A buddy of mine teaches there. I know their open house is next week. Something to think about."

Allen was right. We had nothing to lose, so ventured afar. Barely into the school tour, Matt tugged hard on my arm, stopping me dead in my tracks. "This place feels safe and I like it. Let's find the principal and talk."

Matt approached the first person he spotted with a nametag and we were quickly on the heels of the principal, Mr. White. A teacher pointed him out ascending a stairwell. Our intrepid son wove his way past people, catching up to Mr. White as they both reached the second floor. I was a few steps behind.

"Excuse me sir, but can I talk with you for a minute, once my mum gets here?" He motioned for me to hurry.

Stepping aside from the throngs of prospective students and parents, Mr. White looked Matt in the eye, moving closer to ensure he captured every word. It was hard to block out the cacophony of noise that surrounded us. Matt succinctly and clearly explained his challenges, before declaring that he would very much like to attend this school.

"Matt, I'm impressed with how well you've identified your learning difficulties. That's good information for any school to know. In this school, students with similar learning issues are taught in a specialized classroom, with one consistent teacher. She focuses more on practical life skills, than on the regular curriculum. To be honest, we have absolutely no experience with including a student with a disability in the regular classroom setting."

As Matt's chin started to drop, I steeled myself to intercede. But it wasn't needed. Mr. White cocked his head and said, "You know, that doesn't mean you can't apply. We're always open to trying new approaches and I think we still have some openings."

A beaming Matt thanked Mr. White before making a beeline for the office. The application for regular programming was automatically accepted and enrolment became a reality. A heavy weight was lifted from our shoulders. Exiting these school doors, our lungs filled, expanding our chests with hope.

In the early days I dropped Matt off downtown near my work and he caught public transit from there. After school he either came to my office or took two buses home. On mornings when Matt was slow getting ready, I often caved in and drove him to school. Neil disapproved.

"Susan, you cater to him. Dropping Matt at the school door and making yourself late for work doesn't teach him anything about responsibility. He's capable of catching the bus from downtown and paying any consequences for being late. So don't complain to me about you arriving late to a meeting. You've got to let him fall and get up on his own. But that's my broken record. I'm off to work. Dinner's almost ready for you."

Giving an insipid wave, I tossed a hand towel over my shoulder, ignored dishes waiting to be dried and walked away. This wasn't the time to spark a skirmish.

Neil's goodbye felt icy cold. Maybe we'd pick this up later, but likely not. We'd both be too exhausted when he got home.

I returned to the kitchen once Neil closed the back gate. A chill still lingered. Only when she dropped her pen did I realize that Kate had been silently present during the squabble. She looked up from her homework, strewn all over the table.

"Dad's right you know. You're way too soft on him."

"Not you too! Easy to judge from the sidelines. I'm the one on the frontlines here. If you really want to help, clear your homework and set the table. I'm taking five minutes before we eat." Neil and Kate tag teamed me too often.

Behind the closed bedroom door I sat on our bed, head in hands. I was caught in a vice grip of family strain and needed space to breathe. I knew there was truth in Neil's comments but if I didn't go the extra mile to get Matt to school on time....

The school made efforts to understand and accommodate Matt. They quickly assigned a teacher coordinator, Ms. Jansen, to provide support and modifications as needed throughout his high school experience. She expected him to work hard and put in effort, which he did. Despite growing pains, progress was obvious and Matt was proud. Ms. Jansen approached me on a warm fall day as I waited for Matt after school.

Leaning against my car's door frame she said, "Mrs. Dunnigan, I want you to know that Matt has challenged me in positive ways. I'm getting much more creative, developing modified approaches to the

70

curriculum. It's making me a better teacher." I reached out and gently touched her hand.

"That's music to my ears. Speaking of Matt, here he comes." Laden like a mule with his heavy backpack, he ambled towards us.

Ms. Jansen waved to him before patting the car door and heading back inside. My mind kept replaying her reaffirming comments. There's a chamber in my heart reserved for such encouraging system allies. Their words of endorsement help sustain me in bleaker times.

Matt's muscular and skeletal challenges made it difficult for him to meet the bar of the demanding physical education curriculum. Rather than playing sports alongside his hormone-raging athletic peers, an alternative was offered. Matt became the equipment manager for the junior and senior football teams. He learned about football rules and strategies while fulfilling a valuable role on the team. He helped keep the athletes hydrated, encouraged their efforts and enjoyed being one of the guys on the bus. Along with the players, he had his head shaved as part of the Cops for Cancer fundraiser. Our bald lad was very proud.

One wintery day en route to school, Matt saw a man collapse on the sidewalk. Without hesitation, he directed the bus driver to call 911, hopped off and applied recently acquired skills as a certified first aider. He waited with the man until the ambulance arrived, then headed to school. The City of Edmonton formally commended Matt's actions and sent a copy of the letter to the principal.

The principal honoured Matt's actions by presenting an "Award of Excellence for Service and Leadership." Whether they knew Matt or not, all 1,200 students at the school's monthly assembly got a glimpse of our son's humanity and contribution to a caring society. How many of them would have looked out the bus window and wondered if the man was okay, without acting?

In the spring of grade 10, the assistant principal unexpectedly asked for a meeting to assist with transitional planning for grade 11. She requested that both parents attend. Being the consistent point person when dealing with the school, I was curious why she wanted us both there. I didn't ask—but Matt would have.

We exchanged pleasantries and settled into chairs facing her desk, when the office door unexpectedly opened. The school counsellor joined us, nonchalantly pulling up a chair. Their overly cheery professional demeanour exposed the guise of collaboration and transparency. I scrambled to become finely attuned to their secret radio frequency. The unspoken agenda quickly surfaced.

This was an intensified version of the grade five challenge to our inclusive education path. My brain raced, before the penny dropped for me. Requesting both parents was a divide-and-conquer strategy. I was the intractable adversary and Neil the unknown. They hoped to put a wedge between us.

Stressing their credentials, both professionals spoke about the low statistical likelihood of academic success. They openly scoffed at families who they referred to as "sacrificing their sons and daughters for the dream of being included at all costs." Our recently acquired advocacy training reinforced how the system readily turns to such catch-all phrases, as a diversion to throw people off balance.

Neil and I both bristled with the implication that professional knowledge and authority trumps parental knowledge and perspectives. Neil cleared his throat to speak.

"Depends on what is meant by *at all costs* and who's in the best position to assess that. With all due respect, professional roles are narrow in scope and usually time limited. Parents are the constants—in it for the long haul, appreciating the full picture and having a universally recognized natural authority."

I was buoyed by Neil's comments. Learning that we were united, I expected them to back off. Not so.

Meaningless terms and phrases were tossed around, still trying to disarm us. Looking concerned the counsellor said, "We only want what's best for Matt and his well-being."

"Our sentiments exactly," Neil retorted. They'd struck a nerve. The gloves came off.

These professionals felt emboldened and were undeterred by our clarity. The veil of generalized disdain lifted and our quest for an inclusive education was directly questioned.

"We know you are philosophically opposed to segregation, but help us understand one thing…. How can you dismiss a well-developed educational program that you've never even looked at?"

They'd executed a finesse chess move, while not taking their eyes off us. We were shell-shocked. To avoid shredding our reputation as open-minded parents, we reluctantly agreed to visit the school district's segregated program. Years of extensive professional and personal experience had fine-tuned my awareness of how seemingly simple suggestions can readily lead to the slippery slope of segregation. Fear gripped every aspect of my being, but I chose not to share aloud with Neil.

As parents we share a common view on inclusion, yet have different approaches to dealing with worries. I need to talk matters through. Neil prefers to sidestep, as long as possible. I learned a long time ago to accept this difference. Raising issues during late evening quiet time was rarely fruitful. I'd go to bed upset at leaving the discussion in limbo. I'd hear him exhale a long sigh, before scrolling through TV channels.

My husband typically dealt with important matters when they presented a clear and present danger. Arriving home from work at about 10 p.m. every evening, he was tired, hungry and ready for mindless television, not serious discussions. Weekends were filled with projects, commitments, routines and if lucky, a small shot of relaxation.

The school's hastily arranged meeting was on Monday morning, so there was no relaxation that weekend. Just tense muscles and minds. My biggest fear about visiting the segregated district school was that Neil might be tempted to surrender.

We drove engulfed in silence, swimming in private thoughts and pummelled by waves of angst. I desperately wanted Neil to pull over but refrained from intruding on his thoughts. He needed to process without influence and draw his own conclusions. That didn't stop my brain from silently screaming for him to stay strong and be on high alert. Undoubtedly Special Ed would be presented as a panacea. Keeping my tongue firmly knotted, I refrained from uttering a single word.

With shared trepidation we walked through the school doors. The enthusiastic school counsellor was proud of the school's offerings and how it supported students. Sitting in his office he tried to engage us.

"So I understand you're looking to see if our school could be a good fit for your son."

"Actually, we're wanting to compare what both schools have to offer," I replied. Neil remained silent.

The counsellor slapped his desk with the palms of both hands, smiled broadly and stood up. "Well then. Let's have a look around and we can talk after."

The tour revealed a plethora of non-challenging, loosely structured classroom activities and hallway decor typically associated with much younger children. In short, I was hard pressed to see any educational value. My overall impression was that of filling the hours—floating along, waiting for recess, lunch and home time.

Two particularly memorable features were the well-stocked, bustling candy shop and the small animal enclosure where students learned to care for rabbits and clean their cages. Both were touted as popular with students and focused on teaching job skills. Smiling politely, I kept wondering what was going on in Neil's head, praying that we remained on the same page.

Back in his office, the counsellor eagerly shared a success story. "Why, a student has done so well that she now participates in a regular class at our neighbourhood high school. For the past couple of months, she's been attending morning classes, twice weekly."

Had he forgotten that our son attended a regular high school, full time, five days a week? I dug deep for an appropriate response.

"Bet she and her parents are proud of her bravery. So many coordination intricacies, support considerations and close monitoring required to help her truly fit in. Hope she gets the needed support."

The breadth and depth of this educational chasm seemed to elude him. I couldn't fathom how incredibly intimidating her experience would be. Those mornings transported her from a patronizing, juvenile setting to the biggest high school in the city, bursting with over 2,700 students. Opportunities to fit in with the student body would be superficial and contrived at best. Matt being included in mainstream classrooms throughout his entire educational journey was challenging enough.

Wrapping up, he said, "Openings fill up early so you might want to submit an application for next year pretty quick." Reaching for papers conveniently placed on the far corner of his desk he added, "I have a copy here if you'd like."

I chose my words carefully. "We appreciate you taking the time to show us what the school has to offer. This visit has given us lots to think about. If we're interested in pursuing this option we'll be in touch." Turning to Neil, "Ready, hon?"

Nodding, Neil stood and shook the counsellor's hand. We thanked him and quickly made an exit for the door. I started to breathe once outside.

Neil was quiet as we walked to our car at the far end of the parking lot. I could almost smell thoughts marinating in his skull. It was important to hold back, yet I asked for his impressions as we approached the car.

"You know, I'm glad that we came," he said softly.

Damn—he was still processing! Seeing my face blanch, Neil's face softened and his arm went around my shoulder.

"Susan, even on our toughest days, nobody could ever convince me to consider such an alternative. But now we can say we checked it out, which should silence them. What I saw only served to reinforce that there's nothing special about Special Ed. See, all that advocacy training did pay off," he added with a smirk.

I laughed and gave him a big hug, infusing him with my elation. This stressful experience reinforced our resolve as a couple. Nobody could put a wedge between us, taking the spectre of a segregated education off the table for good.

By grade 12, Matt's adapted physical education curriculum needed a shake-up. The school found low-hanging fruit—helping lead physical education drills in the Special Ed class. This forced association felt natural and right to the system, but not to me. But I was too exhausted to offer a creative alternative.

"Mum, I knew you wouldn't like the idea. But really it's okay. I don't mind. It's actually kind of good because I'll get out of school 15 minutes early each day."

"I don't understand. How come?"

"Well the Special Ed class starts 15 minutes later every morning and gets let out 15 minutes before the rest of the school. It's for their own safety."

"Pardon me? Explain please."

"The hallways are too jam-packed with regular students at the beginning and end of each day. Someone could get knocked down and hurt. See, it's for their own protection."

"Rather than focus on protection, I think it would be better to emphasize courtesy and respect for all. Now those are skills that can benefit everyone. Bet if one of your classmates was on crutches or in a wheelchair, there'd be no early release."

"Oh Mum—just let it go, okay?"

"Will do." I released a long sigh, discouraged that Matt was buying into the rhetoric of protection, rather than respectful inclusion and accommodation.

The stress from years of striving for ordinary experiences within the public-school system was showing in our family. Matt was the first person with a discernible developmental disability to be included in every public school he attended, from elementary to senior high. No wonder we felt depleted of energy and gasping for air—especially Matt.

Nearing the finish line, sweat, exhaustion and stumbles magnified. Great promise dissipated and dark clouds of stubbornness brewed. The dark sky produced a sprinkling of skipped classes in Matt's final year, followed by torrential rain.

In the early spring of grade 12 a rainbow of brightness warmed us. An insightful student recognized Matt's tenacity, submitting his name for consideration at a student-nominated annual awards ceremony. Students saw this annual event as their version of the Academy Awards. Matt was anonymously nominated in the category of Bravery, likely by his friend Will. I had no illusion about Matt winning. The prize was not in being proclaimed a winner, but rather being recognized at a deep human level for being a pioneer on the road less travelled. There was no question—we would attend the awards ceremony.

Awards galore were listed in the program. One category caught Matt's eye—Excels in Sports Outside of School.

Matt leaned over and whispered in my ear, "Steve's bound to win this category. Don't see him anywhere though."

Steve was a gifted athlete by all community standards. He excelled in Special Olympics, at the national level. The sad reality, however, was that Steve was not even on the nominee list. The winner was a popular student whose listed athletic accomplishments paled in comparison.

Shortly after the awards, I was asked to present an overview of our entire inclusive education experience at a public meeting of the Edmonton school board trustees. I consciously strived to ensure a balanced perspective, fostering a commitment to inclusion. I gave an overview of approaches that worked well at each educational level and identified what could have worked better. No blame was laid.

Minutes before my presentation, a parent from the audience wished me luck and commented that she wouldn't be so brave. I assumed she recognized my nervousness and meant bravery in public speaking. Clarity came later.

When closing my presentation, I referenced the recent student awards and the conspicuous absence of nomination for the athlete in the segregated class. I thought it was a stellar example of how segregation, without ill intent, can leave people behind and invisible to their peers.

The next morning, I received a surprise phone call at work from the principal. "Mr. White, is everything okay with Matt?"

"Yes. I'm calling about your presentation last night to the school board trustees. I have you on speaker phone with Matt's coordinator, Ms. Jansen, and the Special Ed teacher." He'd swooped in with his troops. I was flying solo.

His frosty tone and unilateral involvement of other professionals conveyed annoyance and intimidation. Feeling overpowered and potentially under siege, I stalled.

"If you can just give me a moment, I'll close my office door so as not to be disturbed."

I used that opportunity to consciously draw emotional support from advocacy allies. Thinking of their warrior strength sitting on my shoulders grounded me. After a few deep breaths, I sat and picked up the phone.

"Okay, I'm ready, Mr. White. I sense that you have a concern about my talk."

"Yes indeed. One of our teachers attended last night's presentation. He said that you shared things about your experience at our school that were untrue."

"Excuse me, Mr. White. What I shared was very balanced and reflected my experiences. *Nothing* that I shared was untrue." My heart was starting to pound. Turning my head from the phone, I quietly absorbed a few deep breaths to help calm my nerves. The principal pounced.

"I beg to differ. Specifically, you mentioned our annual student awards night and how Steve wasn't recognized. As a matter of fact, he was recognized and loudly applauded at a school assembly."

"There's the rub. What I referenced was the annual student-nominated awards, not a monthly assembly. Out of curiosity, can I ask who recognized Steve at the assembly?"

"Yes, it was his teacher. What does that have to do with anything?"

"A lot actually. I'm sure the students clapped when the teacher mentioned Steve's prestigious national award in Special Olympics. However, the reality is that for the annual student-nominated awards, Steve was not nominated by his peers. It seems he wasn't even on their radar. That speaks volumes to me and it's why I raised it."

"Teacher or student initiated—doesn't matter. You shouldn't have insulted our school." His volume increased and agitation resonated in his voice. I was feeling bullied. Power imbalance or not, I needed to stand tall.

"Mr. White, I was not trying to insult. My goal was to share my experience respectfully and truthfully, from the lens of inclusion. And that's what I did."

"Everyone's included at our school, no matter what classes they attend." This message didn't mirror the Mr. White who welcomed trying a new approach when we first enrolled. He clearly missed my point. So I tried again.

"I'm not the best person to have a fruitful discussion with you on mainstream inclusion, versus shades of inclusion. If you'd be open to it, an Alberta Association of Community Living representative would gladly meet with you to discuss inclusion concerns, issues and strategies."

"No, Mrs. Dunnigan, that is not needed or wanted." His agitation was undeniable. I'd had enough. Time to retreat and replenish my sapped energy.

"Understood. Mr. White, we're getting nowhere with this conversation so I'm hanging up now. Goodbye."

My trembling hand struggled to hang up decisively. Mission accomplished. Emotions bounced off the walls, colliding in the air—stunned, dismayed and elated. I stood tall against intimidation. After 10 minutes I regained sufficient composure to open my office door, hoping nobody would come looking for me. I was still absorbing the ripple effects from every blow and counter attack.

That call was the last time the principal and I spoke. I don't believe that he had malicious intent. Rather, Mr. White didn't comprehend my perspective. An opportunity for deepening understanding through respectful listening was lost and open dialogue was silenced.

Now I better understood what the parent at my presentation meant. She knew something that I didn't at the time—perhaps knowledge gained from her own battle scars. I realized I was brave to speak truth to power. It was my advocacy training and warrior angel army that helped me stand my ground with the system and dare to unilaterally end the conversation.

Matt sprawled across the finish line of high school, too exhausted to raise his head. He marked time, avoided classes and skipped tests Ms. Jansen thought he could pass. As the school year wound down, the only highlight was proudly attending the gala graduation dance, with his girlfriend on his arm.

Ultimately, it was the calendar, not final tests that denoted the end of the arduous marathon. Despite narrowly falling short of achieving a high school diploma, Matt's educational foundation prepared him for the next leg of life's journey. Adventures of adulthood, employment and post-secondary education awaited. Ready or not....

Family Life

Chapter 8: High-Wire Acts

Randomly plucked from the conveyor belt of parenthood, love was our guide. Unwittingly enrolled as high-wire performers, by virtue of seeking *ordinary* for our child with significant vulnerabilities. Intent on tapping his potential, and ours, we stretched and became more agile.

Spellbinding high-wire professionals are perfectly in sync and completely trusting. Performances reflect intensive practice of well-choreographed routines, with safety nets and harnesses, just in case. No such luxuries for us. Neil and I balanced on tightropes and soared high on the trapeze. Nothing choreographed about it. Trial by fire was the norm and rife with risks. Love and commitment softened the impact when balance was lost and leaps of faith fell short.

Relying on every sinew in our fingers, we often succeeded in grasping each other's outstretched hand. At other times we've fallen short or the other hand felt withdrawn—a world away. Like all parents on this perilous route, we've been repeatedly tested.

We desperately clung together through dark falls into seemingly bottomless pits full of venom—judgement, betrayal and victimization. We learned to weave our own safety net to reduce toxic risks.

It was natural that our daughter, Kate, became an apprentice in this family performance. She became drawn to the trapeze, sailing across the gulf. Her keen bird's-eye view of the world came with a price. Neil and I spent an inordinate amount of time addressing her older brother's teetering balance. Our sweet daughter garnered the traits of perceptiveness and independence, while relying on us to be her safety net if she fell. To Kate's credit, she became strong to her core. She has a big heart and flows with life's natural current, not against it—lessons she learned from on high.

For almost four decades our marriage has endured strains, sprains and occasional green stick fractures. Like the mended broken bones of the high-wire athlete, we've become stronger at the point of initial trauma. My personal and professional experience with disability reinforces resilience as universal, in all marriages that survive. We're the lucky ones—many couples have disintegrated under the pressure. Love is at our core, yet at times we've limped along, licking our wounds, sometimes ones we inflicted on each other. What has kept us from breaking is our values and a common vision for our son. It's been a profound, life-altering experience—a shared one, but from differing perspectives.

Our parenting roles are quite traditional. I'm the maternal nurturer, often viewed as too soft, accommodating, naïve and malleable. My innate grasp of Matt's complex layers and swirls makes me ache for societal tolerance and understanding of both his potential and limitations. Neil adopted the deeply entrenched male role—Matt's guide to becoming a man.

Neil's calling in life is that of teacher and Matt has been his biggest challenge. As Dad, he was eager to show, guide and support Matt practically and morally to become a competent, confident and courageous man. Perpetually impulsive and overly enthusiastic, Matt acts first and thinks later. He rarely wanted parental guidance, believing that he understood processes intuitively, was informed by a TV commercial, a stranger enlightened him on the bus and so on.

Neil routinely got frustrated with Matt ignoring his advice. Our child's inability to comprehend risks often landed him in untenable situations. The base of Neil's emotion was firmly rooted in love and he feared for our son's well-being. Many conversations happened in the kitchen, well into adulthood. On this day Neil and Matt had been jousting about what constituted vigilance when crisscrossing the city on buses. Matt ended up walking away in a huff.

"Bye, Mum. I'm outta here!" I heard the front door slam.

Neil whipped the tea towel over his shoulder. "He never listens to me. How can I teach him if he won't listen?"

I stopped washing dishes. "Matt tries to listen, but readily interprets input as being told what to do. Saying *you need to* triggers him. A suggestion versus a directive is best, in theory."

"Bottom line—he does need to listen for his own protection. As his mother you know how explosive his emotions can get. Somehow he needs to gain more self-control." I snatched his tea towel and dried my hands.

"Hon, I'd like that too, but we both know it's far easier said than done. He gets so upset when he perceives injustice. Trying to understand why he's upset is the only way to nip it in the bud. Again, easier said than done."

"Doesn't help that societal fear runs rampant. Too many people jump to conclusions without any attempt to understand. Overreaction, from both the public and police, has become the norm." Always a hot button issue for Neil.

"Sadly, I agree. Empathy and common sense are increasingly rare commodities." Pausing, I added, "And marginalized people pay a huge price."

"Sometimes the ultimate price. The Polish immigrant who was tasered and died in the Vancouver airport in 2007 was an early tragic example. My biggest fear is that Matt will be angry over something minor and get tasered by an overzealous, undertrained cop. Susan, you need to know that if someone *ever* tasers my son, I'd likely end up in jail."

Neil openly acknowledged his nightmare. It resonated with me but went unspoken. Such real risks sat knotted in my gut, a stress ball, too huge to escape from my throat. Pretending to focus on

84

dishwashing, my shoulder wiped leaking tears, while my collapsed face absorbed the weight of his truth.

As a couple, our tightly interwoven values and vision for humanity still left wiggle room for individual perspectives, approaches and sensitivities. Sometimes we'd talk about things and other times, simply accept differences. I recall the day I raised concerns about the negative power of labelling.

"Neil, it bothers me when people say *Williams Syndrome kids*. Rubs like a sore corn, pinching my foot. Definitely prefer *kids with Williams Syndrome*."

"Really that much of a difference or a moot point?"

"Huge difference! They are kids first. The syndrome's undeniably linked to their being, yet doesn't define them."

"I know that," he said with a hint of annoyance. "Still, our annual picnic revolves around Williams Syndrome kids and families. Maybe being a bit oversensitive?"

"Don't go there, mister! Precise words might elude me at the moment, but like that pesky corn, I'll get it out with time." As it turned out, words weren't needed at all. The point was made crystal clear on a family vacation later that summer.

Matt and a peer named Donnie connected and became inseparable during the annual Williams Syndrome picnic. Passing through southern Alberta on vacation the next month, we visited Donnie's family. As it turned out they had plans to travel through Edmonton in a week or so. In the interim, we suggested that Donnie join our camping adventure and they could pick him up at our house the next week. Done deal—no criminal record check, just parent-to-parent trust and sharing of home phone numbers. It was in the days before cell phones.

Over the five days with Matt and Donnie, these two 15-year-old boys were with us constantly. Their diagnostic similarities were

85

evident, but what was abundantly clear was their uniqueness as people. Enjoying the campfire while the kids were washing up, Neil revisited our earlier discussion about terminology.

"Now I get it" he announced with a broad smile. "Intellectually I understood your rationale before, but didn't fully comprehend it. This experience has crystalized the difference. Can't believe it eluded me for so long. Trust me, lesson's there to stay."

We both have fond memories of the Matt and Donnie vacation. Managing swimmer's itch and enjoying their renditions of simple rhyming songs that didn't rhyme contributed to many humorous and insightful moments.

At times I've been pressured to choose a family member's "side" on an issue. But I can't fathom how to do that. My love can't be divided up and proportioned. Vulnerability needs to be bolstered— and sometimes support needs to be felt by all family members. Being fair to all parties is a delicate balance, especially on a brittle wire that's ready to snap. That's when we've courted disaster.

The summer when Matt was about 18, Kate was away at a YWCA camp for an intensive counsellor-in-training program. Neil and I planned a vacation, away from the gruelling drudgery of jobs and endless chores. While Matt was confident that he'd be fine home alone for a week, we didn't share his confidence. Much to his chagrin, we insisted he tag along. Digging in his heels, he nixed our first proposed destination.

"Okay Matt, I give in," Neil said. "So let's go to Grande Cache instead. I hear it's beautiful and we've not been on that road before." Neil desperately needed this break.

After much cajoling, Matt packed his trusty Jump Rope for Heart bag and begrudgingly hopped in the back seat. The first three-hour leg of our trip was flat prairie with little to see. At Hinton we'd stop for lunch, then turn north to discover new terrain, in scenic mountain country.

Matt lacks his sister's ability to go with the flow. Disappointments and inconveniences were being tallied—dull scenery, no animal sightings, too long in the car. As the scenery went from dull to deathly boring, the backseat grumbling consumed all oxygen. Nothing I said helped and Neil was getting more annoyed. Billed as a relaxing break, our vacation was already more stressful than work. Brittleness crackled like electricity. Finally, we stopped for lunch in Hinton.

After lunch, we prepared to embark on the final, more scenic part of our journey. Neil started the car and turned to Matt in the back seat, who was already muttering.

"Matt, the boring part is over. I'm excited to head north to mountains we've not seen before. *But* I've had it with your complaining. So keep a lid on it and be grateful for the chance to get away."

Matt was far from grateful for being conscripted into an unwanted getaway. "No Dad—I'm done! This is *not* how vacation is supposed to be. You guys can stay if you want but I'm leaving. I'll hop the train back to Edmonton. When we walked past the station, I saw it leaves in an hour. Just need food money for the train and taxi to get home."

He jumped out, slammed his door and stood by my open window. With an outstretched hand he demanded, "Mum…money please."

"Not a chance, young man," Neil snapped. "Get back in the car right now. To get a decent camping space we need to get moving. Still have to buy groceries and set up the tent before supper."

"Matt, your dad's right. This has been a boring trip so far, but it'll get better right away. You can help me with groceries later— hotdogs and beans for dinner?"

"No! I'll hitchhike home if I need to!" With that he stomped across the main street walking down the main road, heading east towards Edmonton.

As he walked, Matt kept looking over his shoulder to see if we were following. Neil and I discreetly kept watch in our car's rear-view mirrors. It was like a spy game, waiting to see who would blink.

Neil accused me of pandering to Matt's wishes and temper tantrum. Matt wandered under a foul dark cloud, while Neil felt ignored and irrelevant. I was caught in the middle. It was an untenable situation and our fragile house of cards was about to fall.

"Susan, I know Matt feels like a prisoner being dragged along against his will. God knows we both need a break from him too. So far he's been a royal pain in the ass and calling all the shots. That stops now."

"Let's give him five more minutes to chill, then I'll try to—"

"Stop trying to cajole him!" The valve burst on Neil's pent-up frustration. "If anyone's catching the train back home it's me!" With that, he reached into the back seat, grabbed his bag and swung open the door. "I'll leave the keys. You go wherever you want!"

Grabbing the keys from the ignition, I was in hot pursuit. Neil was determined to avoid me. He needed time and space, not capture. He slipped into shops and hid behind corners as I searched in vain. Matt undoubtedly wondered where we'd vanished. I felt emotionally pulled apart. Matt would have to wait. Top priority had to be sorting things through with Neil.

The train blew its whistle as it left the station. Thankfully no family member was on board. Neil eventually slowed his pace, allowing me to find him. The emotional intensity was such that neither Neil nor I recall details of this flashpoint.

Undoubtedly, we had a heated exchange of perspectives, but stood united as parents. Holding Neil's limp hand, we returned to the unlocked car. After a few minutes of silently staring out our respective windows, Matt found his way back to us. He plunked himself in the back seat.

"So, what are we doing?" Matt asked.

"Going home!" we shouted in unison.

"Geez, no need to get mad at me. I was only asking. Home's fine with me. A long drive—and all for nothing!"

I turned with fire in my eyes. "Matt, shut up! We need peace and quiet." Peace was in short supply that day.

After a few days to decompress we hesitantly ventured on a daytrip. We drove to Innisfail, a small community boasting the Discovery Wildlife Park. We'd been totally unaware of the park until we saw an intriguing ad on TV. It was home to highly trained bears that had appeared in Hollywood movies and commercials. In captivity, the bears roamed on acres of land, within large enclosures.

During a private one-hour tour and demonstration, Ruth, the trainer mesmerized and informed us of bear traits, identification markers, training strategies, bear safety and wilderness precautions. Her love, respect and connection to these creatures ran deep. The tour was entertaining, educational and insightful.

Wrapping up the tour, Ruth identified a photo opportunity for park visitors to sit on a bench, with the black bear from the TV ad standing tall behind. She'd demonstrated training techniques with him earlier. Then she mentioned another option—a picture with Ali Oop. It was the first mention of him.

Ruth swept open her arm, gesturing to our left. Turning, we were astonished to see a massive, dark presence approaching from within his expansive enclosure. Ali Oop was a 1,400-pound brown Kodiak bear. He had starred in many movies including *Dr. Doolittle 2*, *Wild America*, *The Last Trapper* and *True Heart*. His signature role was in the 1999 movie *Grizzly Falls*.

Ruth had worked with Ali Oop for over 20 years and their close bond was evident. His extensive acting experience and training were key factors in allowing souvenir pictures with the gentle giant. The Kodiak stayed on one side of the electrified enclosure, with the visitor facing him on the other.

Ruth spoke clearly and authoritatively. "There's absolutely no reaching out to touch. Just pucker up and Ali Oop will lean over the enclosure for the kiss. Any takers?"

A picture with a giant movie star bear? Matt bounced with excitement. "Mum, I've *got* to do it—please. This will be so, so cool!"

We coughed up $20 for a shot from a Polaroid camera. While I contained my nervousness, Neil found the best spot to take his own picture. Matt stood by Ruth in front of the enclosure. On her cue, Ali Oop stepped forward. Matt didn't understand it was a one-way kiss.

The purchased picture was disappointing, but that was okay. Neil's telephoto lens and photographic skill magnificently captured the kiss. Looking at his shot on our home computer, Neil enlarged it, again and again and again. Chuckling, he called me to have a look.

The decisive moment was captured. Matt had interpreted "pucker up for the kiss" literally. When the bear went in for the lick, Matt went in for the kiss. His lips connected with the bear's tongue. Matt came downstairs to see if his dad's picture was better than the Polaroid.

"Look Matt, take a really close look," Neil teased. He moved his chair away so Matt could get closer to the screen. "You're doing the kissing. Kissing a bear's tongue—now that's certainly unique."

Matt was sceptical about doing such a thing. Neil drew him closer and enlarged the picture until there was no denying. Good-naturedly Neil nudged Matt. "See, am I right?"

Matt repositioned his glasses, triple-checked and blushed, saying, "Well…well…let's just say it was equal."

Neil and I both cracked up at the innocence. Matt quickly added his laughter. No residual brittleness remained from our Hinton trip. Stability had been restored. Who would have thought that a vacation that started off so poorly would end on such a note? The framed picture was destined to become a timeless conversation piece.

Stability during stormy times requires teamwork. In matters of advocacy, I'm typically on duty. Neil has great faith in my abilities, seeing me as stronger than I do. That can leave me feeling besieged with addressing all things Matt related. I usually wait until I'm overwhelmed before asking for his active support. By then my message is garbled and shared through sobs, with hands covering my tear-stained face.

Shortly before securing a condo for Matt, all family members remarked on refreshing strides in his attitude and awareness. Tired system representatives were sceptical, with both Matt and me feeling dismissed before fully formed thoughts were aired. He struggled to translate clear thought bubbles from his brain into coherent sentences. I was scarcely able to get a phrase out in his defence before being interrupted. As if the system knew our intentions and needs better than we did.

Admittedly fixated on his extremely limited finances, our son had some legitimate concerns that merited attention. Angry outbursts became Matt's battle cry for understanding. System representatives wouldn't tolerate his initial blast of emotion, which once expelled, allowed him access to clear expression. I had no solace for either of us.

That's when I turned to Neil, my warrior angel. I can always rely on him when battle fatigue has me gasping for air, on wobbly legs. He rides over the hill in the nick of time—and not a moment before.

"Hon, I need your help. It's always me on the frontline. You're the guy in the background who doesn't say much. The system seems convinced that I'll do whatever Matt wants and you'll go along with me, no matter what.

"That clearly proves they've not been in our heated kitchen debates when we differ on strategies, consequences and impacts." He smiled, but my throat tightened.

"You must admit you don't say much at meetings."

"That's because you can handle it and speak their dialect. Bureaucratese is a whole new language. You really don't want me to weigh in—I'm not the diplomatic one." Again—the smile.

I couldn't hold back the pent-up tears any longer. "I just need a little reinforcement, so people know we're on the same page."

Wrapping me in his arms, Neil tenderly held me. "Tell me what I can do."

"Emailing the trustee with *your* overall perspective would help." I paused to wipe my tears on his sleeve. "In an email earlier this week she questioned if Matt might *manipulate* us into giving him free condo rent. She knows Matt's layers of complexity and that it was a stretch for us to swing a condo down payment. I couldn't bear to respond to such professional naïveté."

The next day, with zero input from me, Neil sent the following email to the trustee.

As Susan has mentioned, we are presently experiencing a significant change in Matt's behaviour with his family. This change that we see is an opportunity for us to encourage him to treat others with more respect and hope that all of you in his life will begin to see these changes as well. We, more than anyone, understand the feeling that "we have seen this before" and it is easy to be cynical. Thanks for your help, advice and patience.

At a meeting shortly after the trustee shocked us by saying that Neil sent an accusatory email and chastised her. Disbelief washed our faces. The agency director who chaired the meeting saw our reaction and would not be deterred from the agenda.

"Sorry folks, with lots to cover we need to stick with macro issues and not get caught in the minutiae. So let's get at it."

If only Neil had copied her on the email, we think the issue would have been given at least a minute of airtime to clarify. We felt bulldozed by the system's needs and sensitivities. Immediately after the meeting, the trustee left on vacation. Holidays turned into an extended leave and we never saw her again. I had no idea what factors came into play, triggering her response. The incident reinforced that the system is sensitive and slaps hard.

As marital partners navigating disability and inclusion we slipped and gained scars, with some residual pain, lasting years. Over time, we've become softer and mellower. Even the jagged edges from our "Vacation Interruptus" gradually smoothed out. From the outside, some things could be perceived as an easy gloss-over. However, looking at a situation from afar and living it are galaxies apart.

Living on the high wire of vulnerability has made our hearts stronger by being tested. We've expanded our capacity for vitality, endurance and resilience. At times our blood has pumped fast, heart rates soared dangerously high and recovery periods were essential. Like high-wire professionals our balancing and daring feats have entwined our hearts as inseparable bodies. Whether balancing on the tightrope or flinging ourselves through space reaching to grip the other's hands, we are unconditionally united.

For years we buried feelings in a shallow grave, close to the surface. Daring to dig up corpses for autopsy didn't feel worth the risk. It's only been recently that we've disturbed the site and dissected pieces, large and small. We can laugh about events with dark humour— nobody was strangled and divorce was averted. Now in retirement mode, reduced daily stress and ample time together facilitated discussions. Topics laid bare, that in the past would have been squashed early. Time's been an essential salve to soothe old pains and resentment.

Candour, understanding and appreciation of differing perspectives now rule—usually. In shakier moments, I turn to Neil for reassurance: "You'll catch me if I fall?"

"…Always."

Chapter 9: Christmas Grows Up

"Mum, it's long overdue." Glancing out the window, I stood at the stove stirring spaghetti. I was busy processing her message, not ignoring it.

"Kate, time to turn on the light. The first week of December and already it's dark before five o'clock."

"I know—don't change the subject." Persistence could be Kate's middle name. She flicked on the kitchen light. The brightness foreshadowed the pending interrogation.

"You've got to tell him. It's not fair to him, and you know it. I'm in grade five, I know and all my friends do too. I even suspected last year. Anyone else in grade nine still believe? No, just my brother. Mum—you listening?"

"Yes and I get it. But it's not as straightforward as you think." It had been a tough day at work and I wanted to cook an easy dinner in peace. I kept stirring.

"Duh, it's easy—just sit him down and tell him. Otherwise he'll always jump up and down when he puts cookies and milk out for Santa. Oh yah, can't forget about the carrots for Rudolph." She rolled her eyes and gave an exasperated sigh before continuing.

"Do you know what Matt's doing while you're here cooking? He's glued to the living room window admiring the neighbour's new Christmas lights. Bet he'll want to show you after dinner. Now that would be the *perfect* time for your talk."

God, she was good at pressuring! Placing the wooden spoon across the boiling pot of water, I turned to face our daughter. "Christmas is still a magical time for Matt. It's not like I'm reinforcing his belief in Santa. I'd never lie or sidestep his questions either. I want him to come to the realization on his own."

95

"Well, that would be never. If you don't tell him he might say something stupid about Santa at school. Then they'd really make fun of him. You sure don't want that. It's embarrassing enough for me. How do I explain it to my friends when they see how excited Matt gets?"

"I'm not falling into that trap about your friends. They know Matt well, so it wouldn't surprise them at all. Understand your point about his peers though. Still, not likely to come up. Excitement usually doesn't kick into high gear until school's out for the Christmas break."

"That's a lame excuse. Come on Mum, what's your real reason?" She leaned against the counter and let silence hang like fog in a mountain valley. Stopping the barrage gave me time to seek my own clarity and gather thoughts.

"Christmas is a special time of sheer joy for Matt. You got just as animated, until recently. If still believing in Santa brings some sparkle to his life, I don't want to take that away. Most parents don't ever have to do that."

Gently she added, "Mum, he's 15. It's time."

"Logic isn't the issue. It's my heart, not my head that's hesitant. Matt's life isn't nearly as robust as yours. He has few friends and no sleepovers or sports to enrich his life. Snuffing out the magic of Santa feels wrong, especially since he doesn't make a public display of it. He's known for years that Santas in malls and parades are imposters."

"Oh, you mean like imposters of the real Santa? Now you're stalling."

I laughed, "That did sound lame." My heart was starting to be more receptive.

"Mum, you always talk about wanting Matt to have a normal life. Believing in Santa is not normal for anyone his age. So here's my *extremely* generous offer. I'll wash every single dish after dinner tonight, without complaint, if you promise to talk to him after dessert."

"All right. You're like a dog with a bone."

"Wonder where I got that from," she said, making one of her silly faces. "Seriously, you can do this, Mum."

"I know and I will. Won't enjoy it though."

During dinner, my head whirled with favourite Christmas morning memories. Our family's tradition was for Santa to leave each member an unwrapped gift in plain sight. My job was to contain impatient pyjama-clad kids at the foot of the stairwell, while Neil did last-minute preparations. First, he started the coffee maker then took his post at the video camera, ensuring everything was ready to capture Christmas magic. Waiting for his go-ahead seemed endless, but we've been rewarded with a treasure trove of recorded memories.

One year in particular always makes me smile. Kate asked Santa for a Starbright doll, as most kindergarten girls did that year. She ran to the prominently placed doll, tightly clutching and kissing it. I turned the switch on the doll's crown to shine its jewelled pattern on the ceiling. Being morning, the pattern wasn't as splendid as advertised, but she didn't seem to notice.

"Katikins, after everyone sees their Santa gift, let's take Starbright into the bathroom and close the door. Her jewels will glow super bright in the dark." Kissing her forehead, I turned my attention to her brother.

Matt had paused momentarily, scanning the overflowing Christmas stockings and gifts, then exuberantly bounded across the room. The video camera captured him enthusiastically arching his back and repeatedly pumping his fist. With a face of sheer radiance, he grabbed the Nintendo. Turning to Neil, Matt spontaneously unleashed a thunderous high five. The heat from their perfectly

97

executed connection imprinted a lingering glow on both faces. Such magical Christmas memories filled my head, carrying me miles away.

"So can we…? Mum, did you hear me?"

"Sorry Matt—guess I was daydreaming. What are you asking about?"

"I was talking about the neighbour's flashing Christmas lights and wondering if we can buy some." Kate caught my eye and winked…as if I needed a cue.

"I didn't notice but they sound nice. Maybe you can show me after dinner. Kate's taking care of dishes tonight so that gets us both off the hook."

Swallowing his last bite of marble cake, Matt reminded Kate that she was on dish duty, then hustled me into the living room. We shared the window bench, admiring how lights can brighten frigid winter nights. When smoke from our neighbour's chimney drifted past, it seemed to make the lights twinkle in the haze. This shared enchanted moment was my sign. I broached the subject gently.

"Christmas will be here before we know it. Bet it's getting exciting at our new neighbour's house. Those three little boys will have trouble sleeping when the big night arrives."

"Oh yah. I remember how hard it was for me to get to sleep. Always hoping to see Santa, but never did." He shook his head and giggled at the image in his head.

"So what about now? Do you really expect to see Santa arrive on a sleigh with reindeer?"

"Nah, not really." Matt shifted his body, leaning a bit farther from me.

"What's changed?"

"You know Mum, it doesn't feel so real any more. Don't get me wrong, I love Santa and whatever he surprises me with."

"You typically get a cool Santa gift, often something you really wanted. But you stopped writing or going to see mall Santas."

"Too old. God, it's been years since I sat on Santa's lap."

"So what's your theory about how Santa picks the right gift and gets it to you?" I looked deep into his eyes.

"Truthfully, I do have my suspicions." A smile wiggled its way across his face.

"Don't keep me in suspense," I said with raised eyebrows, gesturing for him to continue. His tightly pressed lips spurred me on. "Spit it out, my son. I'll gladly answer any questions."

"I kinda think that you and Dad might be Santa. Am I right?" His bright eyes were as big and round as our door wreath.

"You nailed it. Santa is a magical creation. And like magic, he's not real. What Santa represents is joy and love—things parents try to offer their children. Santa wraps love with magic and excitement at Christmas time. Kids usually figure it out as they get older. Just like you did."

"So, I was right after all," he said, sounding very pleased with himself. "And those letters Santa sent to me every year? Were they from you?"

"Your dad always wrote them—with absolutely zero help from me. Some of them were pretty funny. I've saved them all. Do you remember the letter from a couple of years ago, when you tried hitchhiking to school?"

"Sure do. Santa said he thought his beard got even whiter when the elves told him about it. That sure made me laugh. And of course, I had already stopped. Now that I think about it, Santa's signature did look like Dad's."

99

"Your dad has good handwriting—not messy like mine." He smiled in agreement, as he digested the disclosure.

"Mum, I have to ask, does Kate know yet?"

"It's funny you say that. She's recently figured it out too."

"Well, good to know. If she didn't, I wouldn't let it slip and ruin Santa for her."

"Nice to see your thoughtful big brother side showing. That's what Santa's been writing to you about for years." I playfully nudged him. "Sure you're not trying to butter him up for a nicer gift?"

"Now that I know who really wrote the letters, I get how Santa always knew about me arguing with Kate." Matt wagged his finger. "Dad's busted! He'll be surprised to learn that I'm in on the secret…and Kate too."

"Matt, there's something special about knowing. It's like gaining access to a hidden chamber that protects the magic. You now have the responsibility of protecting it, so little kids believe for as long as possible. Do you think you can do that?"

"Absolutely. Those three little boys won't ever hear it from me. It's kinda like I switched sides from believing magic to protecting the magic."

"That's a great way to put it. Trust me, it's still magical being on this grown-up side of Christmas."

"If Kate has kids someday maybe I could write them Christmas letters. In some ways I could be like Santa's elf."

"Who knows what the future holds. Kate becoming a parent is out of our hands." I patted his knee and got ready to stand up.

I paused when Matt extended his arm straight across me, reminiscent of when he was a school crossing guard. He wagged his finger at me and stood up first. Making a beeline to the kitchen, he called his sister. "Kate…want to ask you something!"

Chapter 10: Boxing Day Unhinged

My husband wasn't happy. The cereal topping for his traditional brunch dish was going to be skimpy. Extra cereal hadn't been on my mind, let alone my grocery list amidst the throngs of Christmas Eve grocery shoppers.

"So remind me why we needlessly put ourselves under such stress every Boxing Day—a time when most people get to relax?" Neil growled.

"Because they're my cousins and if we didn't host this annual brunch we'd never see them," I snapped back. Both valid points. I'd initiated this practice because I wanted to maintain contact with my Uncle Jim's family. The year after his passing, my cousins stopped hosting their family's annual Boxing Day open house.

Neil and I first met my reserved branch of cousins when as a young married couple we moved to Edmonton "from away." Residing on the fringe of this extended family, we've never quite penetrated their tightly knit inner circle. Whereas they epitomize properness, planning and preparedness, those traits passed us by.

A few years earlier, Cathy laughingly confessed that she and her siblings initially viewed us as a "curiosity of sorts." Adventuring across Canada on a motorcycle likely contributed to our mystery. Blending our different family styles would be akin to forcing the proverbial square peg in a round hole. Instead of mashing, we opted to stand side by side as equals—mutual respect and appreciation of uniqueness ruled. Clear and aligned in core values, both families genuinely liked each other.

Every Boxing Day, over a meal and too many cups of coffee we talked and laughed, exchanging the highs, lows and twists of our year. Like unwrapping an annual Christmas parcel of family news, my cousins shared routine tidbits, as well as big and small surprises. Neil and I maximized our time to glean what was stale news among the siblings. "Hard to believe you surpassed last year's record for attending Fringe Festival productions—camped out there, perhaps? Wait a minute—surgery? For what?" And on it went.

Preparation for this annual reunion always involved frantic last-minute bustling. If better planners, we could jump right to the enjoyment part. While not in Neil or my DNA, it was a common trait among my cousins.

Both Matt and Kate were prodded to get dressed and tidy their Christmas Day mess. Begrudgingly having complied, Kate saw Matt still on the couch, glued to his new Game Boy, the hot item on every boy's Christmas list that year.

"How come I need to clean up and he does whatever he wants?" she huffed.

Like a drill sergeant I barked, "For the umpteenth time Matt, get movin'! We have company coming and you're still in pyjamas. Go!"

"Five more minutes, Mum, just five minutes, okay?"

The preoccupation with this stupid game was already driving me crazy. Experienced at picking battles, I gave in.

"Okay, but I'm setting the kitchen timer. Your idea of five minutes on Game Boy stretches on forever."

Matt got up when the timer rang. I was impressed, thinking that he'd put down his game and was headed to get dressed. Ambling into the kitchen instead, he gave us a bewildered look.

"Holy smokes, Mum—thought brunch was ready! Why's it still in the oven? Don't want it burnt." When our son learned his annual favourite had almost an hour left to cook the kitchen temperature skyrocketed.

"Geez Dad, why didn't you get busy and put it in earlier? Guests will be coming."

Neil sizzled. "You're damn right they'll be here and you haven't lifted a finger! So get dressed now or say goodbye to your Game Boy."

Shaking his head, Matt grumbled, "Okay, okay, but I need a bowl of cereal first. I'm hungry." The empty cereal box was the final injustice. "Arghhhh! You're both incompetent today and way too bossy. I'm going out—now, like right now!"

A volcano had erupted, spewing thick emotional lava. What little oxygen Matt inhaled evaporated in the heat. We'd been down this dark path before.

He dashed upstairs for his jacket to throw over pyjamas. Close on his heels, Neil and I shut the bedroom door behind us.

"Matt, it's freezing today, minus 30 Celsius, plus the wind chill— skin freezes in minutes!" With no response, I changed tactics. "You always enjoy this visit and brunch will be ready soon. Isn't getting dressed better than freezing and going hungry?"

"Outta my way!" he screamed, ramming into us, trying to get past. Neil's face got that detached look, a sure sign that he was turning to the last resort. He dropped the cloak of Dad and drew on his expertise garnered from decades of teaching non-abusive restraint. He adeptly corralled Matt and hugged our son's flailing limbs. Folding both bodies into one, he lowered them onto the bed. Employing a firm bear hug with inherent wiggle room, he cradled our son's thrashing body and wrapped his legs around Matt's, ensuring mutual safety.

"Matt, I'll release you as soon as you calm down. I promise. We just need you to stay safe inside with us." But Matt's access to rational thinking was slammed shut, like his bedroom door. At times like this, words are almost pointless.

Matt's body squirmed and flexed relentlessly, fuelled by pure adrenaline. After 45 agonizing minutes of contained thrashing, Neil was drenching sweat and on the brink of exhaustion. Meanwhile

Matt's boundless energy gushed through an open portal of rage. Recognizing the futility of his efforts, without warning, Neil released his embrace. Matt leapt to his feet, grabbed his jacket, and sprinted downstairs for the door. Hot on his heels, Neil yelled "Grab hat and mitts by the door." Matt ignored him.

Muscle memory numbly carried my feet down the hairpin stairwell, which I couldn't see through my tears. Neil had done his utmost to keep Matt safe inside, but now our son was racing towards unforgiving winter elements.

When the doorbell rang, it thrust us harshly back to reality. Without breaking stride, Matt changed his trajectory. Turning away from the back entrance he rushed to open the front door for our first guest.

"Merry Christmas, Helen! Boy it's freezing out there. Can I hang up your coat?" In the blink of an eye, his one-track mind had jumped the tracks, catapulting him from furious escapee to gracious greeter.

Looking up from Matt's beaming face, Helen saw me darting into the bathroom in tears. Realizing something was dreadfully wrong, she asked if we were okay. "It's all good," Matt answered without hesitation. "We've had a little family disagreement, but things are fine now." Transformed into the consummate host, he nodded at Neil. "Would you like a coffee? Dad will be making a pot. Mum's just in the bathroom. 'Scuse me while I get dressed."

After dabbing my puffy face and red eyes, I regained composure enough to slink into the kitchen. Matt was already there, fully dressed now. "Sorry I got mad, Mum. Gotta say, you sure don't look ready for company. Not even close to happy."

I suppressed a primal urge to scream, restraining my anger. "How could I be, after what just happened?"

Matt looked perplexed. His struggle to process our family's distress was unmistakable. "Yah, but it's all over now. Just be happy—like me."

"Oh Matt, what felt like a ripple in your day was like a tsunami for us. We're emotionally devastated."

"Devastated? Why? Everything is fine now, really. I'll go ask Helen how she takes her coffee. See, I'm helping."

I cupped my face in search of sanity, then dug deeper for courage. Facing my cousin, family warts were on full display. Neil's emotional exhaustion and defeat were deeply etched on his face. Processing the meltdown trauma silently, Kate faded into the background. When passing her in the dining room, I heard a barely audible sigh. Like a shredded washcloth hung out to dry, I couldn't wring out a drop of energy to console her. That was too often the case.

The doorbell rang again and Matt merrily skipped off to welcome two more cousins. Excitedly he spotted another car pulling up, so kept the door wide open. Letting in the cold blast did little to dissipate the residual electricity crackling in the air. Clandestine sibling glances conveyed an SOS signal.

Our fragility, like fine crystal, was handled delicately and with tact, much like a family tragedy still too fresh to process. Helen, Mary and Alice seamlessly slipped into hostess mode. Walter and Dan kept the atmosphere light and conversations flowing. Each person drew us in from the periphery, gently but surely. Employing their matter-of-fact approach and organizational wizardry, they gracefully, effortlessly and efficiently took charge. The role change was as fluid and comforting as a roadside stream after a sudden summer downpour.

Neil and I were nurtured back to emotional stability, treated as guests in our own home. My cousins made ample coffee, took the meal from the oven, set the table and limited our role to identifying the location of utensils and extra chairs. An unspoken agreement kept topics light while good-naturedly engaging Matt in conversation. Kate, embarrassed by our family's full exposure, kept a low profile.

An avid cat lover, Alice chatted with Matt prior to the meal. "Scooter's purring so loud on my lap, I might need to get a hearing aid," she teased.

"He's even louder when he snuggles me at night. You put me right to sleep, right Scoots?" Matt beamed as his favourite cat leapt from Alice's lap to his.

"Okay Matt, I know you're a big movie fan," Walter said. "So tell me, what latest ones are worth spending my money on?"

"Hmm, been lots of good ones lately. Saw a great movie last week. But first they showed an amazing trailer. I'll be first in line for tickets when it's released. Don't want to spoil it, so let's just say if you like action you're in for a treat!"

"I'm an action and suspense fan," Dan said. "What's it called?"

"It's called—um, um—oh gosh I forget!" Matt slapped his thigh in laughter, then his face contorted and tears filled his eyes. Residual tension broke the dam, gushing down his face. "Don't know why I'm crying…"

Gently Mary chimed in. "Oh Matt, you're not the only one around the table who can instantaneously transform laughter into tears. I'm good at it too." Smiling heads nodded and someone passed Matt a tissue. Kate subtly motioned for him to tuck the used tissue up his sleeve. She was slowly returning to the moment.

Neil and I gradually shed the tautness in our muscles and minds. Equilibrium appeared on the horizon and enjoyment filled earlier cracks of despair. Buoyed by the food, company and conversations, Matt kept vigil over me. His eyes divulged concern, struggling to understand my emotional flatline. For him, the "little family disagreement" was over, so didn't define an otherwise good day.

As Helen and other cousins bundled up for the elements, we exchanged long heartfelt hugs. "See you next year—same time, same place!" was echoed all around. Everyone smiled at the truism.

The darkness that shrouded us had given way to light, but what a lightning storm while it lasted. The experience reinforced that loose-knit family bonds can be deceptively resilient and strong. As the incident left no residual battle scars for Matt, he has no associated memory. We shake our heads in wonder.

Chapter 11: Spring Cleaning

Winter insisted on one last icy bite—ignoring the calendar that already declared spring. But hot banana pancakes filled our bellies on this frigid prairie morning. Neil's delicious fare helped prime the cooperation pump. Chores were on the day's agenda.

Matt with his hollow leg was tackling a third *saddle blanket* pancake that overflowed the plate. Now age 12, Kate still placed special orders. She requested a pancake shaped like an elephant, with huge ears and a long trunk. Neil didn't disappoint.

"Pretty impressive, Dad. Looks like you still have your magic touch." Kate licked her lips in anticipation.

"Dad's always made the best pancakes ever," Matt added between bites.

The day was off to a nice start. Blustery weather made it a perfect day for the kids to spring clean their rooms. With brunch wrapping up, it was time for me to stipulate the rules of engagement.

"This process can go smoothly and quickly, by following simple rules. Remember, the hallway isn't a storage area, focus on your own work, no hiding items and no dismantling furniture." My eyes locked on Matt when delivering my dismantling comment. "You should be able to get it all done in about an hour. I'll inspect to ensure you've covered all the basics, then the day belongs to you."

"Easy-peasey, I can have it done in 20 minutes," Kate said.

"Don't think so. Stuffing things into your closet doesn't count. And be prepared for me to check. You'll need to vacuum too."

"Okay, a half hour then. I'll probably be done before Matt even gets started."

I gave her a sharp look. "This is not a contest. Stick to your own work—that goes for both of you."

Pushing back from the table Kate adopted a sprinter's stance, counted to three, then darted upstairs. Getting our youngest on track was easy. The eldest would need more clarity and supervision.

"Okay Matt let's go upstairs and develop a game plan." He downed his last bite, patted his full belly and unexpectedly belched as he stood. "Oops, sorry. Can't believe that popped out." He chuckled all the way to his room.

In our modest one-and-a-half-story home, kids' north- and south-facing bedrooms were joined by a compact hallway. Glancing into Kate's room, I saw she had already made her bed. She was hell-bent on having everything done in a half hour.

Matt opened his bedroom door and we both took a step in. There wasn't much point in going farther. A grenade couldn't have made a bigger mess. Piles of clothes littered the floor, the stuffed hamper was piled sky high and last week's crumpled bed sheets obliterated the desk and chair.

Stale movie popcorn overflowed his bedside table, joining the empty pop cans that poked out from under his double bed. Rolled up movie posters were bursting the confines of the designated corner wastebasket. At 16, our son held his first part-time job at the Paramount Theatre. He loved it, but the perks were a mixed blessing.

When tidied, Matt's room was a sight to behold. He'd chosen emerald green walls, with a tan feature wall. The two-inch tan trim demarcated the beginning of the sloped white ceiling. The wall trim was perfect for thumbtacking movie posters—all new or recent releases. Glossy movie posters enlivened the walls with a plethora of colours and vibrant images. The tacked posters kissed each other, consuming every inch of valuable real estate. The current crop promoted animated Disney movies, action movies, thrillers and superheroes. He loved them all. The line-up changed at least biweekly as new releases came out. Scanning his room revealed new posters, balanced on the sheets atop his desk.

"Oh, Matt... You picked up more after last night's shift?"

"Oh yah. Got some good ones too. Don't worry I'll figure out which ones need to go. It'll be hard though. Like 'em all."

"That's always the issue. But you can decide that tomorrow, not today. You've got a lot to tackle already. Doing laundry would be a first step to finding your floor."

"I'll take my hamper down now before Kate beats me to it. Then I can fill up for another load later. Good thinkin', right?"

"Sure, but hustle. I'll wait and can help plan if you want." Teenagers are notoriously messy but Matt was a leader of the pack.

He quickly returned, proud that one load was already in the laundry. Without prompting he rushed about filling the hamper with random pyjamas, shirts and socks.

"Okay Matt, you seem motivated. Before I turn to my work, let's pull up your bed covers." I moved the edge of his comforter from the floor. This adjustment awakened Matt's bedmate, his beloved cat Scooter. Poking his head from beneath the pile, Scooter stretched and prepared to leave his nest.

"Oopsy—sorry Scoots! You sure are being a sleepyhead today." Matt kissed Scooter's head, gave him a rub and let him escape downstairs.

"Matt, I'm following Scooter's lead and will leave you to it. Your empty garbage can sure can be filled up a few times. You know where the garbage bags are. I'll check back in a bit."

"Don't need to Mum. I'm on it. Tell me when the washer's done so I can put in another load."

In less than an hour, Kate was done. The only remnant was popping a load of laundry into the dryer, once Matt's was dry. In the meantime, she grabbed a book and sprawled on the living room couch.

Neil and I enjoyed a coffee at the kitchen table, having taken a short break from our projects. It was reassuring to hear Matt moving about in his bedroom, directly above us. Since progress was being made, pace was not a worry. Then an unusual noise caught our attention, like something heavy being pushed.

I put my ear to the adjoining heating vent that carried sound well. Turning to Neil I shrugged my shoulders. "Don't know—he's mumbling about something being hard."

"Well he's *roominating* and that's hard work," Neil said.

I swatted him with a tea towel. "Not your best pun my dear. Still, I'd better check."

From the stairwell landing, I saw our proud and sweaty son in the upstairs hallway. He was accompanied by his mattress and box spring.

"What on earth are you doing? You know nothing goes into the hallway."

"Oh Mum! Won't be here long—just part of spring cleaning my room. Doing a good job and wanted to vacuum under the bed. This got in the way."

"For heaven's sake, Matt! The vacuum hose extends under the bed, so no need for this. How's everything else coming along?" I couldn't get a glimpse into his room as the bed blocked his doorway.

"Going good, but a lot of work. I'll let you know when the bed's ready to go back. It'll be too hard to get both pieces back in by myself."

"Make it snappy. You've already been at this for a couple of hours. Everyone has work to do. Not fair if we have to stop our work to help you." With good intentions Matt typically took on too much, got overwhelmed and relied on the troops to restore a semblance of order. Maybe this time would be different.

Matt continued to squeeze in and out of his room bringing up a hamper of clean laundry and grabbing a bottle of spray cleaner to wipe his furniture. We were grateful for his efforts but eager to see more results.

Kate was still reading her book when I brought her clean laundry up from the dryer. "Your last job is to fold and put it away." She reluctantly marked her page and headed upstairs with her hamper.

From the landing she bellowed, "Mum! Why'd I get stuck with such a jerk brother? Mum...I can't even get into my room!"

I'd forgotten about the mattress and box spring. Neil was working on a project in the garage. Before asking him to help, I needed to intervene in the sibling squabble that was sure to ensue. I joined Kate and her hamper, on the stairwell landing.

"Omigod—Matthew, show your face right now! Kate, go get your dad. A mattress, box spring and now your *bed frame*—all jammed in the hallway? There's not an inch of space for you to get out of your room or for us to get in. This is unbelievable...."

Peering from a narrow opening in his bedroom doorway Matt said, "Didn't mean to... The bed frame had dust and a bit of spilled Coke so I decided to give it a good clean. A bolt was loose and when I tried to tighten it, it fell out. That made it easier to take them all apart to clean properly. Look at them—they're a lot better now." His face searched mine for signs of why I was upset.

With a straight arm, I shot my hand palm upward. "Stop now—not one more word. You need to pull the bed frame pieces and the box spring back into your room. That way Dad might be able to get in to help you reassemble everything." Dejected, I sat on the stairs and waited for reinforcements to save the day.

Between Matt and Neil, bed components were eventually reassembled. Meanwhile I started dinner and Kate set the table. Matt followed his dad's advice to make his bed quickly before I came up to talk with him. The room was relatively in order, except for one thing that was very out of place. We'd upgraded to a newer TV the week earlier and after much negotiating our eldest inherited the old.

"Matt…why's your TV on your bed? That's incredibly unsafe."

"Mum, it's okay, really. It's not on the edge. Gonna try it on my desk instead of the dresser. Just be there a minute. I'll move the posters and hamper off my desk to make space. You *always* worry way too much."

I cupped my hands and caressed my defeated face. "I'm too tired to argue with you. This room cleaning project's eaten up most of the day. Your dismantling antics ate our time too. Speaking of eating— dinner's ready in five minutes."

When I reached the bottom stair, Matt's bed creaked. Instinctively my whole body spasmed. Time suspended for a split second, before the kitchen ceiling shook with the thud. Momentary deathly silence was followed by a thunderous cry of anguish. I closed my eyes and took a deep breath. The day had started off with such promise, now this….

Thankfully the bedroom carpet cushioned the blow. The TV repairman shook his head in disbelief and made no promises. Miraculously he repaired the damage, prolonging the TV's life for another year.

Extending a handshake Matt sincerely said, "You, sir, are a true professional. I promise to never, ever do that again."

Nor did he—at least, to the best of our knowledge.

Chapter 12: In the Wings

Kate became an unwitting expert on waiting. Like an accomplished, well-loved background singer she rarely got the spotlight. Centre stage was routinely occupied by her brother.

When she did elbow or charge her way to the forefront, friction and angst were at the ready. Electricity routinely sparked and zapped during the teenage years.

"Stop, Matt! I'm goin' to the corn maze with my friends and you've got no say."

He shook his head dismissively. "Not a good idea Kate—way too easy to get lost. Quite sure the police helicopter searched for people there last year."

"You're nuts! Where do you come up with this crap?"

"Not crap—might've heard it on the news. Bet the police have statistics."

"Then prove it, you jerk! Uh-huh—go ahead. You can't, right, right?"

"Enough—both of you!" I wailed. "Kate, get ready to go. Matt stay put—definitely no need for statistics."

Matt's obsessive tendencies permeated daily family life, tingling under Kate's skin. Intellectually understanding was one thing; accepting the onslaught was another, especially when she was targeted. Still, I glared at Kate for stirring the pot.

Kate's background role was not intentional. Realizing this does nothing to reduce my sense of guilt and regret. When one family member's needs are prevalent, time and energy are in short supply for others to soak up and thrive. This is particularly true with siblings. It's hard to pinpoint when this insidious pattern began.

Matthew was four when Kate was born. He adored her, as much as she adored him. From babyhood throughout her preschool years, it was a love fest. They were inseparable, daily basking in each other's love and attention. Matthew took his role as big brother, her protector, very seriously.

While he tried to keep Kate tightly wrapped, metamorphosis was unfolding. His little sister was once like a caterpillar—fuzzy, familiar and manageable. Before his eyes she was transforming into a butterfly—delicate, colourful and hard to contain. Her emerging independence scared him. Matt was acutely aware that his younger sister had as much freedom as him, and was gaining ground fast.

Developmental differences became apparent early on. Where Matt was delayed, Kate excelled. In the playground, Matthew, at age seven, struggled to cross three monkey bars, with assistance. I cheered his efforts, boosting him up while trying to stay clear of his dangling, frantically kicking legs. His fine fingers struggled to retain a grip on the steel bars. My arms ached from his repeated attempts.

Kate, only three years old, insisted on trying too. Holding her as high as I could, she leapt out of my arms, seized a bar and crossed the whole length with ease.

"Mummy, hold me so I can turn around. I wanna go back the other way too." And she did, lickety-split. Matthew watched in amazement, with his feet firmly planted on solid ground.

Enthusiastically she shouted, "See Matthew, that's how you do it! It's not hard." Kate inherited her dad's athleticism.

My cheerleader role became subdued. "Good job my love! But that's too high for a little girl. You'd be hurt badly if you fell."

"I wanna do it again. Matthew can watch me. It's really fun!"

"Nah, let's go sweetheart. There are lots of other things you can both do. Look—nobody's on the teeter-totter."

116

Without a fuss she moved on, while chattering about how she loved swinging from each bar. Matthew was ready for something less demanding. What took great effort for him reaped little visible reward, whereas for Kate it was the polar opposite. Kate was confident, strong and fearless. Plain for all to see.

Playgrounds are supposed to be fun, not a place where one child's fun is hampered to prevent another from being embarrassed. Nor should it be therapy, yet there I was, routinely propping up Matthew, encouraging perseverance and muscle development. I was on a teeter-totter of my own.

By age five, Kate was already carving her unique niche in the world. She showed an early penchant for being both independent and silly. Mrs. Zucuski, her kindergarten teacher, made a surprising comment during our spring parent-teacher interview.

"Kate's doing well academically and is a sweet girl. As you know, she has a slight tendency to be headstrong. Guess that's to be expected since Matthew gets most of your attention."

Taken aback, I replied, "No reason to worry about her. Kate's fine and gets her share of attention." But was it her fair share? Not really. She was vying for attention in her own way. Matt's undiagnosed multiple challenges were pervasive. At an early age Kate grew accustomed to being second in line, sometimes embarrassed and controlled by her well-intentioned, but misguided brother.

Kate's blessed with spunk and revealed it in countless ways. Never one to tolerate bullies, she learned early to stand up for herself and others, including her brother. During a recess in grade one, Kate and her friend were marvelling at Crystal's new hairbrush. Its hollow handle was filled with water. The girls loved spraying their hair with this magical brush.

From the corner of her eye, Kate saw her grade five brother approaching a bully, who was teasing another kid. At that point in his life Neil often good-naturedly described our pencil-thin boy as "a hockey stick with hair." The bully quickly shifted his focus to the easier target, Matthew.

Kate did not hesitate. "Crystal, Crystal—gimme your brush, quick!" Racing across the playground Kate slipped between Matthew and the much larger boy, standing as an impenetrable barrier to bullying. Dwarfed in size, she matched the boy in resolve.

Calling upon her most authoritative voice Kate yelled, "You leave my brother alone!" Armed with her secret weapon she repeatedly pumped the hairbrush handle, spraying the bully's clothes. With dampened clothes and spirit, the shocked boy stepped back. Just then the school bell rang and peace was restored.

Given Matthew's loose joints, sports options were limited. Swimming was always on the agenda, while soccer was the only team sport our son was enrolled in. With Neil teaching karate, it was natural to enrol both kids in classes at some point. At nine years old, we enrolled Matthew. Karate's focus on self-improvement, not competition, offered a natural pathway to health, fitness and friendship. He valiantly tried to control his uncoordinated body, stay focused and ignore distractions. Sirens from the nearby fire station called his name. Matt willingly participated in karate class, while Kate watched from the bench. She repeatedly asked to start classes and learned some drills by osmosis.

"Five years old is still young, Kate. Maybe after your birthday." It's all about trade-offs and living with the refrain of "just wait." When we did enrol Kate she was a natural. No surprise, she zipped past her brother, as in all things physical. This didn't go unnoticed by Matt. Sustaining focus was hard and his interest waned, so he stopped. Kate excelled and continued for a number of years. In hindsight, holding her back did little to benefit either child.

Mrs. Zucuski was right about our girl. She slowly cultivated an obstinate streak in response to being second fiddle. Inheriting stubbornness from both Neil and me, she wove strong threads into a long steel braid.

Kate endured more than her fair share of childhood injustices, while Neil and I juggled work, home and budgetary pressures. One such pressure was the dreaded back-to-school preparations. They always sapped my time, wallet and energy, long before the first school bell rang. Enticing "Back-to-School" ads promoted high expectations and overspending that I couldn't match. With payday at the end of the month, first-day-of-school outfit shopping was always a last-minute affair.

The year Kate was going into grade six, I was pressed into shopping with both kids, as Neil was delayed getting home. We arrived at the mall late Monday afternoon on the Labour Day weekend—a recipe for disaster. Clothes shopping wasn't a big deal for Matt so it seemed easiest to address his shopping first. Alas, it wasn't fashion, but his perpetual distraction that consumed our time.

Finally, we reached the girl's department, where the racks had been well picked over. At age 11, Kate had clear ideas of what she did and didn't like. Any outfits that appealed were out of stock in her size. Matt's patience dissipated by the moment.

"You're taking way too long, Kate! Mum, buy whatever you want for her and she'll just have to wear it. I'm tired of waiting and waiting. Let's go!"

"Go 'way, Matt! Mum, why did we need to bring my stupid brother anyway? You got his stuff first—always do. Took forever too! Finally it's my turn and he wants to go already. Just ignore him."

"Stop—both of you! Matt, go wait by the entrance—we won't be long. Kate, I'm sorry we got such a late start for your shopping. Check another rack. Time's getting short so you'll need to quickly find something here or in nearby stores." Unfortunately, my timeframe was a half hour off.

The store's public address system blared "Attention shoppers. The mall will be closing in 10 minutes." I'd forgotten that shortened holiday hours were in effect. Shopping time had rudely been snatched from under Kate's nose.

"I'm so sorry Kate, but you need to decide and fast." The only item in her size that she remotely liked was well beyond my price range. She refused to settle for anything else from the slim pickings.

"Then our only option is to come back after school tomorrow to check other stores." A heavy message for both the sender and receiver.

"Attention shoppers, the mall is now closed. Please bring your purchases to the nearest checkout."

Kate sobbed her way to the car. I tried to put my arm around her, but she shrugged it away. Can't say I blamed her.

Kate vividly recalls Matt wearing new clothes on the first day of school. She wore last year's tear-away pants and a souvenir T-shirt my brother had recently sent from the Maritimes.

Never a follower, Kate had no interest in aligning with girls she dubbed "the fashion police." She was confident in her own choices. However, like all kids she looked forward to marking the first day of school with a new outfit. We did get her a new outfit the next day, but it was too little too late. That hurtful memory festered for years.

The silent family expectation was for Kate to contribute, understand and accommodate more pressing needs, typically involving Matt. Inadvertently left behind, unattended and waiting in the wings— waiting to be noticed, get attention, be protected and reassured. Waiting in vain for her turn to come first. As Kate got older, she begrudgingly understood why Matt took so much of our time and attention. She was experienced at fading into the shadows. One such occasion was the memorable Boxing Day that came unhinged.

Resentment ruled the day well into early adulthood. As a teenager, Kate deliberately provoked Matt, in retaliation for him being overbearing. She jabbed then hightailed it to her well-concealed hiding spot in the basement. She always chose her timing well—the few minutes between Neil leaving for work and my return home. I was routinely greeted with Matt's fuming grievances after a gruelling workday. Kate made an appearance once Matt cooled down. She's divulged her secret hiding place, but I still struggle to pinpoint the location in my head.

Where I was embroiled in protecting and advocating for Matt, Neil tried to balance the scales towards Kate (always Katie to him). In childhood he'd lived in the shadows of an older sibling with serious chronic health issues. Life-threatening matters gulped his parents' time and energy before ultimately consuming David's life. Neil related to our daughter's plight, while living the parental reality. Neil wanted to break the poke-and-retaliate cycle, so he took Kate to lunch. He hoped to skim off the top layer of her thick protective armour.

"Katie, you're smart enough to know that with Matt's challenges and vulnerabilities he needs our family's love, understanding and support. Without it he could well end up like that homeless man over there—destitute and abandoned. You're empathetic and know something went horribly awry in that man's life. Share some of that kindness and understanding with your brother, especially when it's hardest."

"Yah, I know. I really do. But Dad, I *hate* being his sister. It's embarrassing. He thinks he knows everything. Telling me what I can do with my friends and where I can go. It's so unfair and I can't let him get away with it. He makes me so mad...a lot."

"You're right and I get it more than you realize. Remember, I lived under the shadow of my sick brother—your Uncle David. He could do no wrong, routinely got me in trouble and was a nagging thorn in my side. But while he lived, I was his protector, just like you are deep down for Matt. First-hand, I know it's incredibly hard standing in the shadow because your brother takes up all the light."

Understanding didn't ease the emotional sting. Kate grew more sullen and angry, particularly with me. How could she not? At a counselling session I was asked to apologize to my teary-eyed girl. Hard as I tried, I couldn't comprehend *what* I was apologizing for. Neil understood, but it completely eluded me at the time. To survive emotionally I processed family dynamics strictly with the pragmatic side of my brain. This self-protective measure served as blinders, shielding me from recognizing Kate's emotional angst. I barely managed to cope with being overwhelmed. Meanwhile, our vulnerable daughter felt abandoned and emotionally wounded to her core.

Kate once reported a knife incident in an altercation with Matt. For years afterward, I was sceptical about it and blocked out all details. Kate reminded me. She had used his precious Zest soap without permission. The "Zestfully clean" ad jingle reinforced that it had prized properties.

An angry Matt spouted, "Can't believe you'd do such a thing! You'll need to buy me a brand-new bar."

"Ah, no that won't be happening. It was the only soap in the tub so I did *nothing* wrong."

Kate started to walk out of the kitchen. Her dismissal of what Matt perceived as a grave injustice propelled her brother into a rage. He grabbed the closest item on the counter—our large chef's knife.

"You get back here or you'll be sorry!" Kate saw the knife, ran and Matt chased her. She found sanctuary by bursting into the bathroom, where the babysitter was sitting on the toilet. Slamming the bathroom door—which didn't have a lock—stopped Matt in his tracks. Who would have thought that the family rule of not opening a closed bathroom door would provide much-needed sanctuary?

I suspect Matt slammed the handle on the edge of our kitchen counter, as an outlet over his indignation and rage at Kate's soap violation. That's likely when our favourite knife mysteriously got a broken tang. With his pent-up rage released, he could breathe and decompress.

The babysitter never mentioned the incident, but Kate did the next day. In true Matt fashion, he loosely recalled being really mad. He had moved on. I tried to convey the seriousness of his actions and potential danger. But it was lost on him.

"Just wanted Katie to listen. Sure wouldn't have hurt her—you *both* should know that. She's my sister." After a pause, "Still think I should get a new soap though."

Kate concedes that Matt had no intention to stab her. Intentions aside, the risk was real. Matt's threatening behaviour while in a tornado of rage could have ended with unintended consequences. All it would have taken is a simple stumble. Stretched taut well past overload, my thoughts could not go there.

As a survival mechanism I downplayed the gravity of the incident with Kate. I stressed intention versus behaviour and even questioned if she exaggerated the incident. It was self-preservation and denial on my part, plain and simple. The broken-tanged knife will always serve as a reminder of times when I had no answers or protection to offer.

As a family we kept patching the ruptures, salving sore spots and struggling to find equilibrium for all. Kate endured a baptism of fire with flames fuelled by her brother. Amazingly, Kate learned to walk across hot coals and emerged as a confident young woman, with a strong values base. With time I've come to truly appreciate the extent of her contributions, sacrifices, patience and empathy.

Sorting through childhood memorabilia, I found the felt marker note that high-school-aged Kate taped to Matt's door the morning he was leaving for Olds College.

Matt have a blast at college. I knew if I woke you up you'd kill me. Well have fun. Be safe. Call all the time. Respect everyone. Keep clean (that includes ur room). And go to class on time! Love Ur Sis, Kate XOXO

When travelling in Australia with her future husband, Robby, the year after high school, they scraped by. Kate relied on her ingenuity versus empty wallet to find creative solutions for family Christmas gifts. Matt was not forgotten. Given his fascination with transit systems, Kate mailed bus-related information—brochures with colourful pictures, travel options, route maps and schedules. Matt was duly impressed.

The jagged edges of Kate's resentment gradually rounded and smoothed as she matured into adulthood. The process accelerated when she gained her own perspective as a mother.

Kate earned deep emotional scars and well-rooted trigger points with Matt. However, they're overpowered by forgiveness, empathy and unconditional love. Kate excels at reframing past traumatic situations, injecting humour to wipe away clinging cobwebs of resentment.

"Hey Matt, remember the Christmas when you gave me a McDonald's gift certificate, then quickly stole it back and used it yourself?" Matt blushed and looked away with a smirk.

"You know you still owe me, right? A $5 gift certificate from back then won't cut it now. I'll want a combo meal, upsized of course."

Matt nodded and turned to his young nieces. "Girls, it wasn't nice of Uncle, but I admit, it is true."

"Done deal then. And I've got witnesses," Kate added, pointing to all family members around the table.

"Girls, you might need to remind Uncle Matt that he owes me some McDonald's food sometime." An angelic preschool duet of "Okay Mama" made Matt beam, as he tousled his precious nieces' hair. Baby Zoe silently watched from her highchair—too young to be counted as a witness.

As Mother's Day approached, Matthew proudly announced that he'd be bringing two gifts to our family's Mother's Day dinner.

"Really, how come?" I asked.

"You know I usually don't buy Kate anything."

"Naturally."

"Yah, but now that she's had a third baby…well I thought she deserved it. I've wrapped both presents really nice. I'll text you pictures right away."

The pictures showed gift bags, beautifully overflowing with colourful tissue. One bag said "Mum" in large print. The other bore the caption "Best Mother Ever." His text identified that my bag was on the left and Kate's was on the right.

"Yes Matt, got the pictures. Nicely presented gift bags." Teasingly I commented, "If I read your text correctly my bag on the left simply says *Mum* and the *Best Mother Ever* bag is for your sister. You sure that's right?" His response caught me off guard.

"Well yah…. After all, you've got to admit Kate's turned into an amazing mum. With three little girls to look after, of course that makes her the best mum ever. Kinda surprised you didn't get that."

"Point well taken." My heart glowed, revelling at his insight.

Little did Matt know that his heartfelt depiction of his sister's motherly love was the best Mother's Day gift he could ever have given me. While he marvelled at Kate's stellar parenting, I was

125

impressed with her increased awareness and sensitivity to her brother's vulnerability.

Viewing Kate in a new light, Matt began turning to his sister when troubled or anxious. He began to listen, sometimes heeding and other times dismissing input. Typical of what we all do.

Kate learned to adeptly and smoothly follow her brother's disjointed conversations. Stream-of-consciousness flow often aborted by mid-sentence derailments. Unrelated thoughts often leapfrog, storming the forefront of Matt's brain and escaping from his mouth.

"Hey Kate. What a difference! That heater you loaned me is awesome. It's keeping my place toasty warm."

"Oh good. Comes in handy during this cold snap. Lots of people rely…"

"I miss you Kate."

"What…what did you say?"

"I miss you."

"Well Matthew Dunnigan, that took me by surprise. Don't ever recall hearing those words before."

"You're probably right…. Certainly wouldn't argue it."

"Robby and I just talked about inviting you to dinner this Sunday. You'd go home a little hairier though."

"Ah, why?"

"Think about it. Besides the girls, both dogs and the cat haven't climbed all over Uncle Matt for at least a week. They'll send you home with remnants from the snugglefest. Our family motto is: *No outfit is complete without pet hair.* It's the price you pay for being part of this family."

Without a doubt, Kate has embodied humour, courage and empathy to claim her rightful place on centre stage. She now comfortably shares the spotlight with her brother—overshadowed no more.

Relationships

Chapter 13: Forsaken

Some memories, like this one, are seared into my brain. The day had been uneventful, until the mailman arrived. His sole delivery was an innocuous neatly printed envelope, addressed to Neil and me. I recognized the return address in the corner, but the exquisite penmanship identified the sender. Such envelopes from my cousin, Rose, typically contained an invitation to a social event or a card marking a special occasion. Much to my surprise, this held a handwritten letter.

Like a powerful earthquake, the message sent seismic shockwaves that rocked our world. Neatly printed ominous words coalesced into a formal notification. Stunned, I reread it. My aunt and cousin were banishing our immediate family from their lives.

A torrent of tears drenched my face and reaction was visceral. Disbelief and anger did a frantic tango. My tightly tensed diaphragm restricted air flow. Rattled to my core, this was a direct hit at home and heart. Ostensibly, it was about a bicycle. For Neil and me, the letter represented an inevitable conflict about values, expectations and relationship parameters. The bike was the flashpoint.

Matthew was to be the sacrificial lamb—the ultimate punishment for clarity of voice. Beautifully scripted words slashed the relationship we'd trusted. Evicted from their lives, the pain pierced, like a dagger. I later discarded the letter—as if that would ease pain. Particularly jagged messages etched in our psyches eventually smoothed, as two decades evolved into three.

Serendipity had led to the nurturing of this familial relationship, which began with good intentions all round. My family heritage, both maternal and paternal, is firmly rooted in Saint John, on Canada's east coast. My paternal side stayed put, while my mother's siblings, all older, had ventured much farther afield. I'd only met my mother's siblings a few times when growing up.

In our first year of my marriage, a career opportunity resulted in a move from the Maritimes, to Neil's hometown of Edmonton. All of his immediate family still lived in the area. Coincidentally, Edmonton had also become home for two of my mother's siblings and their families. Decades before, my gentle Uncle Jim had adventurously headed west as a young man, settled down and raised a reserved, self-reliant family. Much later, my Aunt Grace, her husband, Orville and daughter, Rose followed suit, after Uncle Orville retired from Canada's foreign diplomatic service.

Rose grew up during those diplomatic postings, attended boarding schools, never married and remained deeply devoted to her parents. Intelligent and well educated, she chose to remain at home, supporting her parents to maintain the comfortable, sociable lifestyle they enjoyed. The Edmonton move reconnected them with Uncle Jim and strengthened valued family bonds, after years of living abroad.

Family lifestyles varied dramatically among my mother's siblings and their families. We'd grown up isolated from each other's family units, with limited opportunities to bond as extended family. In Edmonton, my aunt's home became a hub for all things social. New additions to the group, Neil and I were warmly welcomed and contributed our uniqueness to my maternal extended family.

Aunt Grace and Rose exuded aristocracy and were quintessential social conveners. Painstaking attention to planning, etiquette and timing were immaculate, with fine dining assured at all events. Years of embassy life and a clear sense of propriety filled every crevice of their existence.

Meanwhile, well-grounded Uncle Orville sat in his wing-backed chair smoking his pipe. With a wry smile he watched his wife and daughter fuss over details. Whenever he felt they were going a bit overboard, he'd shake his head and say "For God's sake you two…." His warm-hearted rebuke always restored balance and made us chuckle.

After a year in Edmonton, family members, far and wide, were delighted to hear that I was expecting our first child. The pregnancy heralded the beginning of a new generation for my maternal side of our Edmonton extended family.

Neil and I reminisced about childhood memories of nearby grandparents and their positive influences on our lives. Sadly, our child would not have that privilege. Nor would my gracious aunt and uncle have biological grandchildren in their lives. This generational void gave us pause. After much consideration, we decided to offer a precious gift, done in good faith, grounded in love and respect.

One evening late in my pregnancy I raised the subject around their dinner table. "With Neil's parents deceased and mine in the Maritimes, our child won't experience growing up with ready access to loving grandparents. So we are hoping you'd like to assume the honorary roles and titles of Grandma and Grandpa." Looking at Rose, I added, "And of course we'd like you to be Auntie."

The family enthusiastically accepted, bringing joy to all. True to character, my aunt and cousin seized their roles with great zeal. Sadly, my Uncle Orville's cherished role was brief, as he died when Matthew was a mere nine months old. It had been his gentle chiding that initially helped keep my aunt and cousin's well-intended exuberance in check.

I recall the baby shower hosted at their home. Neil's family and my cousins gave typical gifts. As I folded the wrapping from the last present, Rose discreetly slipped away to retrieve her family's gift. She returned moments later, wheeling in a high-quality formal baby carriage, filled with meticulously wrapped gifts. The crowning touch was a beautiful European "fur pocket" for Matthew to nestle in during strolls around the block. It was a work of art. A skilled seamstress, Rose handmade all aspects, including the exquisite monogrammed initials, MJD. All guests, including myself, were in awe. Guests politely took their leave shortly thereafter.

Over Sunday dinner, when Matthew was still a newborn, Rose made an announcement. "Susan, I've decided that I will buy all of Matthew's clothes for his first two years."

"What? That's…well that's incredibly kind and unexpected. But really, it's not necessary. After all, it's just part of parenting." Overwhelmed, I didn't know what else to say.

"No, I want to do it and it'll save you the expense. God knows, raising a child will be expensive and this should help. That's it though. After that you'll assume responsibility." Rose was emphatic—the matter was not open for discussion.

Neil and I grappled to process this proclamation. Lying in bed that night Neil broached the issue. "It's a magnanimous gesture—one that makes me uncomfortable. Once this gets started it'll be hard to dial anything back."

"I know. Been thinking the same thing. Rose has already spent lots on Matthew. Given her good job, she has the means to go into overdrive buying clothes. As a mum—especially a new mum—I'd like to be the one who decides what to buy for my child and when. In some way her mind-boggling offer deprives me of that. Jeez, now I sound ungrateful."

"Don't beat yourself up over it. We weren't really offered much say in the matter. Mixed blessings take many forms." Neil leaned over and kissed me goodnight. My head whirled for hours, before finally drifting into a restless sleep.

Clothes galore came our way—enough to clothe quadruplets. I recall laying baby Matthew on his fur pocket to take pictures. Although not expected, guilt demanded proof that all outfits were worn, before the next batch arrived. I wrestled with Matthew's flailing limbs, hoping naptime could be postponed until all attired his body—even if just for a minute or two. Garments had exquisite

European stitching and details, fit for a prince and befitting a much finer lifestyle than the modest one we lived.

After Uncle Orville's death, a dreaded sense of being beholden slowly took root. Family dynamics had shifted, almost imperceptibly. The relationship with my aunt and cousin began to insidiously weave a silky, invisible web of attachment. Weekly Sunday dinners and ongoing material generosity unintentionally stressed our lives.

Although we didn't weave the threads of expectations, we contributed to its spread, by virtue of meekness and silence. It was me, more than Neil, who hesitated to openly address mounting concerns and risk damaging a valued relationship. A colossal mistake.

Inevitably, every Sunday something impeded us from arriving on time, looking our best—violating social expectations close to their hearts and orderly lifestyle. A far cry from our hectic, disorganized and unpredictable lives. Hanging by a thread, we juggled home, work and financial pressures, coupled with growing concerns about our young child's developmental delays.

Dinners were routinely kept warm in the oven, as our scheduled arrival time came and went. We excelled at coming up short, on a weekly basis. "Arggghhh! Neil—I need you, now! Matthew's spilled milk all over his best shirt. Can you change him into this spare? Hopefully it'll pass inspection. I'll grab a backup, in case there's another spill. Dear God, let the last load of laundry be dry." Before running to the basement dryer, I glanced at the clock. "Damn, we're late—per usual."

"Hello my sweet boy," a beaming Aunt Grace said, as she rose from her chair. Matthew flew into her outstretched arms. We were forgiven, for the moment.

My cousin busily retrieved the dinner from the oven before returning for her greeting. When Matthew released Auntie from his bear hug, Rose's eagle eyes locked on his shirtsleeves. "Oh my goodness, you're sprouting! Susan, that shirt's really too small. I'm surprised he's still wearing it." Judgemental or not, it stung.

I relayed the spilled milk story, but resented the compulsion to explain myself. "Actually, the sleeves *do* still cover his wrists, so it's fine for a bit longer. He's definitely going through a growth spurt, so you're right, its days are numbered." My messages felt dismissed.

"Good thing I found a great sale yesterday so picked up half a dozen new shirts. Come on Matthew, let's get you a shirt that fits you properly." Neil and I exchanged glances. Shirt failed inspection.

Matthew continued to be showered with Grandma and Auntie's love and attention. He was well past his second birthday, yet unsolicited gifts kept coming.

"Don't worry about it, Susan. I thought this outfit would look so cute on him—and see, it does."

Early warning bells that had long sounded in the distance were closer and discomfort rumbled in our bellies. Debt was being tallied with invisible ink. We increasingly felt deep in the "balance owed" column. Thank you, thank you, thank you rolled off my tongue until too numb to form the words. Such simple words sounded insipid and shallow, yet fiercely lashed my psyche. Golden handcuffs of gratitude kept me indentured.

My relatives had the means and desire to indulge Matthew, so for them doing so was not an issue. Neil and I would have gladly provided for our child. However, our working-class standards for what clothes fit or matched fell far short of expectations. Hence my aunt and cousin always stepped up before us, eroding our natural parental roles. Undoubtedly, given good intentions, they never saw it in that light. As differing values and expectations surfaced, resentment took hold. Conflict was inevitable.

At one Sunday dinner we brought exciting news. Instinctively, I braced myself. With an uneasy gut, I blurted, "We're happy to share that I'm pregnant."

133

The room imploded with the gravity of the message. Wide eyes and straightened backs announced the reaction. Rose's eyebrows raised and her jaw dropped before finding words.

"What? You're expecting another child? But you've expressed concerns about Matthew's developmental milestones. He needs all of your attention." Rose looked at her mother, who cast her eyes down and neatly folded the napkin on her lap.

I reminded myself to take a breath. "Another child won't deter us from addressing Matthew's challenges." Squeezing Neil's knee under the linen tablecloth, I added, "We're confident in his ability to share our attention."

Aunt Grace looked up and said, "We thought you were only planning one child."

That got Neil's attention. He'd momentarily been watching our boy blissfully race a truck across the living room carpet. "No, we had no definitive plans one way or the other. Matthew knows our good news and is excited about becoming a big brother."

"Oh," Aunt Grace said. She then reached for her napkin and dabbed the corner of her mouth. In the name of politeness and fact gathering, she asked "When are you due?"

Conversation halted and digestion took a major hit. The sounds of knife blades scraping against fork tangs echoed off the walls, accompanied by chewing and breaking bread. Stone cold silence screamed disapproval.

I highly valued these family ties, so ignored disquieting signs that we'd moved into uncomfortable terrain. We tried to appease without stepping on toes or compromising our values.

As I advanced in pregnancy, Rose suggested that Matthew was old enough to have Friday night sleepovers at Grandma and Auntie's. I remembered such special sleepovers with my grandparents, so had no objections. Rose picked him up after work on Friday and returned him later Saturday morning. All parties enjoyed this new weekly routine. A favourite childhood *Matthewism* was from one such sleepover.

"Did you have fun at Grandma and Auntie's?" I asked one Saturday at lunch.

"I did. But Mummy, poor Auntie fell out of bed last night. Glad she didn't get hurt."

As it turned out, Matthew squirmed relentlessly in Rose's bed, which she kindly shared when he slept over. To get some shuteye and still be readily available in case he awoke, she crawled out and slept on a mat beside the bed. When our son awakened to finding Rose on the floor, he didn't ask how she got there, just if she was okay.

During one wintery sleepover, Edmonton was struck by an unexpectedly severe snowstorm. Rose was well past the usual hour for returning him home. There was no answer on their home phone. An hour late turned into two-plus hours. Police were telling people to stay off the roads and citing numerous accidents. With still no word from Rose, I paced. Worry etched deeply into every muscle. Eventually her car pulled up to the house.

I hugged our boy long and hard. They'd gone shopping and bought a beautiful snowsuit that could serve Matthew well into the next year. Rose didn't think to tell me of her shopping plans. I was not mad, just incredibly relieved. Rather than understanding why I'd become worried, Rose appeared offended.

"For heaven's sake Susan, I'm a good driver and would *never* let anything happen to Matthew. You should know that."

"Agreed. But you don't have control over the horrific weather conditions and other drivers. It's never fully in anyone's control." The message was interpreted as criticism. Her departure matched the iciness of the roads.

Matthew was a freshly minted four-year-old when our darling daughter, Kate was born. No big fanfare this time. More in keeping with Dunnigan practices we hosted a celebratory open house, welcoming friends and family who popped in and out all afternoon. As we proudly showed off our new dark-haired beauty, her whirling dervish brother was never far away. He mingled with everyone, seeking out his new sister every few minutes to give her a hug and slobbery kiss.

At one point I recall approaching Rose, with Kate in my arms. "Would you like to hold her?"

"That's okay. There are lots of people here waiting for a turn. I'll get Matthew. He needs my attention more." She turned away and went off to find him. Her words rippled through my body, resting in my heart.

Baby Kate disrupted Grandma and Auntie's world that revolved around her older brother. Neil and I naïvely thought our new precious gem would quickly wiggle her way past their blinders and become another apple of their eye. Until then tensions quietly brewed and Matthew's Friday night sleepovers continued.

The final straw came after one such sleepover. "Bet you had fun with Grandma and Auntie. What'd you do?"

"Auntie helped me go up and down the street on the bike. It was fun."

"Bike? What bike, Matthew?"

"*My* bike in their garage. It's not for bringing home—'cuz I already asked."

Neil and I talked about this revelation and were united on the issue. Matthew was *not* ready for a bike. The thought terrified us on many levels. Loose joints, lax muscles and balance issues were bodily factors that over time he could master. Coupling this with his developmental delays and impulsivity, the freedom of a bicycle was a recipe for disaster. We wanted him to have a bike, but not now. The timing needed to be of our choosing.

We settled on a plan. They were my relatives and I did not want to jeopardize the relationship. The sensitive situation required both clarity and diplomacy to minimize hard feelings. Neil would be with me in spirit, but I needed to be at the helm of this mission. I called and asked to pop by for a few minutes to discuss something.

"Yes, I'm fine. It's just something niggling at me that I'd rather discuss in person, rather than over the phone." We arranged a time.

I sat down but declined a cup of tea or coffee. I knew full well that my trembling hands would convey my nervousness. Now—to inject confidence in my voice. Thinking of Neil standing beside me, I hesitantly pulled words from my throat, coaxing them from my lips.

"Neil and I were surprised when Matthew shared that he has a two-wheel bike in your garage."

"Yes, we got him one," Rose said, sitting ramrod straight. "We saw no harm. After all, it's of good quality, from a neighbour's garage sale. Didn't think we had to ask permission." Aunt Grace leaned back, so I leaned in. I wanted this to be cordial.

"We appreciate your good intentions, while having some concerns."

"Concerns? Why?" Rose's tone felt confrontational and tension filled the air. I needed to deliver a clear and focused message. My reluctant voice of parental authority balked at being called upon. Stage fright or not, now was the time to speak.

"Matthew's challenges with balance and impulsivity are the primary issues. He lacks the basic motor skills and maturity to safely graduate to a two-wheeler…for now." My pounding heart resounded in my ears.

"Actually, we've been practising for a few Saturdays now and his balance is improving. And of course, I'm holding onto the seat," Rose chided. Aunt Grace remained silent.

"We have no doubt that you'd be very cautious. But the other issue is more personal." Drawing upon inner strength, I carried on. "Learning to ride a two-wheeler marks a significant developmental milestone. For Matthew it will be a huge achievement. As parents that's something that we'd prefer to take the lead on."

"So what are you saying?"

"We're fine with you keeping the bike here for future use, once our boy gains more bodily control and maturity. In the meantime, Neil and I want to determine the timeline and do the running alongside him. We hope you understand."

"Well thank you for telling us in person. Are you sure you don't want some coffee before you go?"

I kindly declined and left. Within the confines of my car my whole body shuddered, releasing pent-up adrenaline. I exhaled a long sigh of relief, started the car and headed home. I thought the hardest part was over. It hadn't even begun. We'd unexpectedly wandered onto an overhanging mass of hardened snow at the edge of a mountain precipice. Unable to hold the weight of our convictions, the cornice gave way without warning.

Rose's letter was confirmation of our fall from grace. The banishment was unilateral, decisive and delivered a lethal blow. Astonished at abruptly being outcasts, we could potentially have worked it out, if the severed relationship was adult to adult. However, it directly involved an innocent—our young son. Kate was still on the sidelines.

Matthew didn't understand why he didn't see Grandma and Auntie anymore—how the hell could he? I didn't understand. Scars became deeply carved into hearts. It changed everything.

Minimally, the severed ties puzzled other family members, but Neil and I chose not to engage. My mum was befuddled by the sudden change. I simply alluded to an unexpected rift. I would never taint the relationship with her only sister, nor put her in the position of taking sides. Sides are rarely black and white. Vantage point, time and distance play huge roles in recognizing shades of grey.

During our phone calls my mother innocently updated me on family social events Aunt Grace and Rose had hosted. Each utterance poked at painful wounds. My innocuous responses didn't encourage, while rapid-fire thoughts ricocheted within the confines of my cranium. "Stop rubbing salt in my wounds! Your innocent grandson was unceremoniously banished—from Prince Matthew to abandoned orphan." The safety valve between my thoughts and mouth had to work overtime.

Thankfully my other Edmonton cousins steered clear of the conflict, not snipping any family ties. As my deceased Uncle Jim would have wanted, they initially carried on their family's ritual of an annual Boxing Day open house. Invited to the upcoming event, we decided to attend. Three months had elapsed. Grandma and Auntie could employ avoidance strategies—or not—as they saw fit. I consciously chose not to waste energy by trying to keep Matthew at our side.

As soon as he saw his much-loved Grandma, Matthew ran over to her. She greeted him with "Hello my sweet boy," and smothered him in kisses. Watching from afar, we saw that she was torn, while not wanting to encourage him. After a few minutes our young son wandered back to us. Neil and I thought maybe we'd get a post-holiday call or letter wanting to discuss patching things up.

Eventually an olive branch was extended—an invitation to their home for tea. Politeness and vague references to misunderstandings ruled, while gritty matters of substance went untouched. Sidestepping and avoidance was a recipe for festering, not healing. Being gun-shy, we chose not to put our children at risk of a second rejection.

Our tale of forsaken relationships is not an uncommon societal story—lines drawn in the sand, with varying perspectives of right, wrong and assignment of blame. Still, if only we'd been brave enough to speak our truths, address warning signs and stay rooted during skirmishes. Perhaps a tragedy could have been avoided or survived, without fatalities.

The reality is that Matthew's robust, yet delicate connection with Grandma and Auntie was shattered. Thankfully he has no recollection of his early preschool love fest and what was ripped away. Although he paid the ultimate price, none of us went unscathed. Family relationships were altered forever—a loss for all. Aunt Grace died bereft of the joy that her honorary grandson once bestowed upon her. Nor did she get to experience the love of an honorary granddaughter.

After her mother's death, Rose and I mutually reached out, to grasp a dropped thread of family connectedness. Wounds have healed and forsaken relationships have been forgiven. Shedding scabs from old wounds, we both acknowledged that clear, reciprocal communication could have salvaged relationships and enriched lives. But there's no turning back the clock.

Chapter 14: Unconditional

The initial spark ignited in our backyard, when our kids were young. It had been our turn to host the freshly minted annual Dunnigan picnic. Free-flowing laughter and conversation crossed three generations—all stemming from Neil's nuclear family of seven kids.

Fifteen years Matthew's elder, Martin took the time to engage his elementary-school cousin. Their relaxed banter focused on topics like animated Disney movies, superheroes, pets and bike riding. The smiles on their faces were contagious and touched mine. In turn, I passed it on.

Two weekends later, after arriving home from grocery shopping, I noticed a manila envelope poking out from our mailbox. Its large cheerful letters identified the intended recipient as Matthew.

I plunked groceries on the counter and the envelope on the kitchen table. Matthew was busy playing with his sister while Neil was preparing dinner. Quickly putting refrigerated items away, I shouted over my shoulder, "Matthew there's mail for you. Come see."

He scampered down the hallway with his little sister in tow. Matthew stopped short at the sight of the envelope, with his name boldly printed in a rainbow of colours. We all gathered around, curious about the contents.

"Mail—for me? This is the first mail that's ever had my name on it. Who's it from?" I'd already looked so knew this was a welcome surprise.

"Check out the upper corner," I prompted. "That usually tells you the sender and their address."

Pushing glasses over the bridge of his nose, Matthew peered closely. It took a moment to absorb the information. "Really—Martin? It's from my cousin," he said, clutching the envelope to his chest. He began jumping up and down on the balls of his feet as if his legs were made of springs. "I wonder what it is!"

"Only one way to find out, but you need to stand still first," Neil said.

Putting an encouraging hand on our son's shoulder, Neil produced a letter opener, demonstrating how to hold and insert it, so as not to damage the contents. "Now you try."

"Hurry, Matthew. I want to see too," Kate said. She wiggled in front of her dad for an unobstructed view.

With vibrating hands, Matthew held the envelope, slowly cutting along the glued edge, with gentle coaching from his dad. His nimble fingers reached in and extracted a single sheet of craft paper. Colourful cardstock toucans, meticulously hand-cut were glued to the sky-blue paper. This surprise was a follow-up to the picnic discussion about Disney characters.

The accompanying note said, "Matthew, seeing these goofy guys made me smile and remember our nice talk. I hope you like them." It was simply signed, "Martin." Delighted, Matthew bounded from room to room, half skipping in his unique fashion. Martin's kind and thoughtful gesture warmed our hearts. After months of display on the fridge, the precious toucans were filed in the childhood memorabilia folder, the keeper of many fond memories.

One sunny afternoon a few summers later, Martin and his girlfriend made an impromptu backyard visit while out bike riding. Like a gentle breeze, their stop reignited that tiny spark of connectedness. As the couple's relationship developed, so did the bond with Matthew. The small ember grew brighter with each encounter. When Martin's work gave him a cell phone, Matt was a frequent caller. My reminders to avoid calling during work hours went unheeded. The calls didn't seem to bother Martin.

"Don't worry about it, Auntie Susan. If I'm busy I put it on silent and let it go to voicemail." Contact increased to many times weekly.

One Saturday morning Matt and I were eating breakfast at the table. Munching his last bite of cereal, he stood up, dialled the phone, stretched the long cord and sat back down beside me.

I hadn't said a word, yet Matt shushed me as the phone rang. "Hi, Martin. Just checkin' to see what's up this weekend."

"Well, hello Mr. Dunnigan. It's funny I was just thinking about you. Janine and I plan to try out a new burger place downtown. We could pick you up around noon—that is, *if* you like burgers."

"Oh Martin, Martin…you know I do. You're crazy, Cuz! I'll be ready and watching out the window." After Martin and Janine married, Matt joining them for weekend lunches and sauntering around town expanded into evening coffees and weekday dinners.

"I won't be home for dinner, Mum. Meeting Martin at his work and goin' to their place. Janine asked what I'd like. She's an awesome cook and I've got so many favourites—hard to choose. They sure do spoil me…and must admit, I like it." Beaming, he hightailed it off to catch the bus.

Matt's teenage angst was latent, protracted and carried gale-force winds. Vulnerabilities, rash choices and curiosity drew him to evening bus rides through the seedier side of town. One weekend Martin dropped by to discuss the concerns that haunted our dreams. Looking Neil and me in the eyes, Martin gave us the priceless gift of an unsolicited promise. "I need you both to know that I'll never abandon Matt." Not hollow words, but a resonating lifetime commitment, laid wide open. The purity of Martin's message shot like an arrow directly into our hearts. He has our family's complete trust, with absolutely no fear of betrayal.

When Matt was a teenager, Martin tragically lost a biological brother—far too soon. What started from a single spark when Matt was a child developed into a unique relationship between cousins. Matt became Martin's brother of the heart, despite the age difference. Martin deeply appreciates his cousin's struggles and vulnerability—up close and personal.

After starting a family, Martin and Janine still ensured space for Matt. He proudly wore his honorary title as Uncle Matt for their two daughters. For years he routinely tagged along for family outings, swimming lessons and watching soccer games.

Typical of all brotherly relationships there are clashes and trigger points. Sometimes healing time is needed before gingerly re-engaging. Matt has inflicted many bruises on Martin's heart, hurling angry, hurtful words without regard for the timing or environment. Such considerations are blocked from Matt's brain in fiery moments.

Anger and associated emotions dissipate as quickly as they are spewed. It's disheartening when Matt behaves like a jerk, takes advantage of Martin's big heart and then gets offended when his cousin draws a line in the sand.

"Oh Mum, that was last week. He made me mad. *Definitely* don't want to talk about it. Martin just needs to get over it."

Eventually someone reaches out, they meet over coffee and initiate repairs. Their strong alliance is built on a bed of coals. Glowing embers can mesmerize and warm, or scorch if unexpectedly spit from the bed. Sometimes flames erupt, with burning tongues of rage. At other times the firebox smoulders and fills with dense smoke. On such smoky occasions they've always found their way out of that darkness, wiped the soot from their pants, taken a deep breath of fresh air and stepped forward.

Martin's introduced Matt to colleagues, friends and neighbours, all of whom have been very welcoming to Matt. Our son speaks about hanging out with "the Greeks," the nickname fondly given to a neighbour and his cousin. These men have invited Matt out socially, offering both friendship and a firm handshake of respect—more threads of community connection facilitated by Martin.

A man of great integrity and compassion, Martin acts according to his own moral code. Surviving turbulent times always provides renewed perspective and a deepened appreciation of his cousin's complexity. If only Matt could reciprocate with a fraction of Martin's tolerance and grace. A loyal guardian, Martin unwaveringly advocates for and supports Matt. One day we met over lunch.

"Auntie Susan, Matt has such a big heart. Yah, he can be stubborn and unreasonable sometimes. Truthfully, people can say that about me too."

"Oh, Martin, it's hard to escape a deeply embedded family trait. Must say I am concerned about how Matt takes advantage of your deeply generous nature." I forced myself to expel the remaining phlegm from my throat. "And he always expects you to pick up the meal tab. Matt's so proud of those rare times when he treats you to a coffee—as if that makes it all square. Wish he was more conscious of your wallet."

My nephew shrugged. "I can handle it. The context for Matt's life is pretty dismal compared to what he sees flaunted on TV shows and ads. No wonder he gets frustrated. Occasionally I do buy him a few groceries or badly needed socks. In fairness, he doesn't expect it. I can't imagine living on his paltry budget."

"Couldn't agree more. As Mum, trying to keep clear boundaries is so much easier said than done. Sometimes what he needs is incredibly basic, so like you, I buy him something. Then I'm labelled as enabling."

"I hear ya. I recently got a call from the agency supporting Matt. Their approach is more hardline than mine, but I appreciate where they're coming from. Apparently, Matt told Nicola that I don't think they're doing a good job and the like...."

I almost spit out my coffee. "Oh, I'm familiar with variations of that scenario. He can be wily, trying to pit us against each other to get something. I'll hear things like, 'Mum you're the only one who thinks like this. Even Martin thinks you're overreacting.' I try to take it with a grain of salt and not take the bait. Doesn't always work though."

Smiling, Martin said, "When Nicola confronted me about what I allegedly said—according to Matt—I invited her to consider the source. I think she got it."

I laughed aloud. "Couldn't have said it better myself. Matt seeks leverage to the best of his ability. It's incredibly easy to get reeled in—the voice of experience talking."

"Auntie Susan, Matt's helped me through some tough times. Whenever I need him, I can always count on him to be there. You can't put a price on that." Martin sipped his coffee.

"Have no doubt, Matt would readily die for you. He doesn't mean to burn relationships, yet once flames get fanned.... Unexpected blustery winds can disrupt calmness, whipping embers into an inferno."

"And that's what makes it oh so interesting with Mr. Matt." Martin flashed a broad grin. "Have no fear, I'm prepared to fight any blaze, with him *and* beside him."

Ah, can't put a price on unconditional.

Chapter 15: Being Uncle Matt

My quiet evening had been hijacked by impulsiveness and *Matt logic*. After an unprecedented police station visit with our son, I was eager to salvage what time remained. As we scampered across the parking lot, Matt pleaded for my phone to call Martin.

"Matt, let me settle in the car before I rummage through my purse."

"Okay. Just know that Martin would be happy with how things worked out."

He was particularly antsy and I didn't know why. Even buckling up my seat belt seemed like a protracted process for my eager lad. Matt plopped the purse in my lap, eager for the phone. My scowl prompted him to return the purse back between our seats.

"Like I said, give me a minute. Why the hurry?"

"Because I haven't talked to Martin since this morning. I need to keep in close touch 'cause his life is going to change any day now. You know he's like a brother to me."

"Yah, I know—a brother and cousin rolled into one." I handed him the phone, silently bid the police station adieu and headed for the tranquility of home. Matt dialled three times but got no answer.

"I knew it! Betcha the baby's on its way. I'm gonna find them."

"First off, there could be lots of reasons he's not available in the span of a whole two minutes. And secondly how would you find them?"

He ignored me, already too absorbed in his mission, calling local hospitals. The third call provided the needed information.

"Got it! They're at the Misericordia Hospital—in the maternity wing. Forget about going home. Turn around—we need to get to the hospital right away. I'm so excited!"

I was conflicted. If I ignored his pleas and drove the final blocks home, he'd head out on his own. New parents want to bask in the newfound beauty of the world, perhaps with immediate family, but that's it. Matt's elation would be such that he'd miss any cues about needing to give the family private time to rest and rejoice.

Capitulating, I pulled over, called Neil and shared our revised plans.

"Alright Matt, here's the deal. We won't stay long and you'll have to wait until we're home for something to eat." His hungry belly might help keep the visit short.

Before the car came to a full stop in the parking lot, Matt jumped out and bolted to the hospital's front entrance. When I reached the lobby, he waved a prized blue note with the room number, pointed towards the elevator and started speed walking. Technically he heeded my reminder about no running in the hospital. However, nimble feet barely skimmed the floor, as if walking a corridor of hot embers.

"Found ya!" he delightedly declared to a beaming new family unit.

"Hi Matt—welcome to the party! Should've known you'd be one of the first arrivals. What do you think of our precious little bundle?" Martin proudly asked.

Joyfully Matt gave two thumbs up, shook Martin's hand and congratulated his glowing wife, Janine. He marvelled at the inherent beauty of their firstborn—a daughter. Congratulations were extended to Martin's mother and sister who had arrived mere minutes earlier. Matt's always been fully embraced by Martin and his family. Still I was glad that the babe's grandma and auntie had the chance for first hellos before our arrival. With immediate family members on their way, a short visit was in order.

"Yah, bet you're surprised that I found you so fast. Got a good head for things like that—I'd make a good detective." Matt tapped his head with his index finger.

"Definitely a good detective, Matt. You've always had a great nose for directions and things like food," Martin teased.

"True, true—you got me there, Cuz," Matt guffawed, slapping Martin on the back.

Matt welcomed the gift of gently holding and cradling baby Anna. One could almost feel him immersing her with love. He talked sweetly to her, saying she had really good parents, even if her dad was a *goofball*. He winked at Martin, then gave Anna a welcome kiss on her forehead. My reminder about getting home to feed his grumbling belly hastened our goodbyes.

The next morning at breakfast Matt arrived in the kitchen looking refreshed and pleased with himself.

"Looks like you had a good night's sleep," I commented.

"Sure did. Had a wonderful dream about baby Anna. It was her first day of school and I got to hold her hand and take her in. Mum, I'm wondering, do you think I could ever get to do that?"

"Well the first day of school is very special. Parents usually save that treat for themselves and the child. Dreaming about it was a bonus gift that floated your way. You'll be able to hold that special feeling in your heart forever."

Crowned with the honorary title of Uncle Matt, our son spent lots of time with the family. He'd gladly have jumped in front of a bus for Anna and later her younger sister, Maggie—even in front of his favourite driver Norm's bus.

One day shortly after Maggie was born, Matt called Martin's mum, looking for his cousin. Isabel shared that the family was there but visiting with her in-laws. Naturally he asked about the girls.

"Oh they're great. Anna's doing a puzzle with Martin and Maggie is snuggling her great-uncle Bob. Can I get Martin to call you in a bit?"

After a pregnant pause, Matt responded. "Auntie Isabel, can I ask you an important question?"

"Sure. What is it, Matt?"

"How come Uncle Bob gets to be a great-uncle and I'm a plain uncle? I'm not trying to be rude, but it has me curious."

Isabel explained it was a generational title and had nothing to do with Matt's greatness as an uncle. With that clarified, he was fine with Martin calling him later.

Martin and Janine always opened their hearts and home to Matt. The arrival of their children enlarged their circle of love. Matt was still included as a natural extension of their own family. As the girls grew, they learned how to clearly and respectfully help Matt understand boundaries. Becoming more independent, they didn't want to be picked up or have their hair tousled. Their messages were always delivered with kindness and love.

As they grew older, the girls dropped the uncle title but it still resonates in his heart, spoken or not. Having these sweet girls in his life opened a chamber in Matt's heart. It stretched and ballooned love in ways he didn't know existed.

Matt's capacity for loving nieces amplified exponentially after his sister Kate made him an uncle in the true sense of the word. Sadly, the expansion did not happen automatically or swiftly. Matt officially became an uncle at a low point in his life. Although living with an encouraging roommate, Matt increasingly dismissed opportunities to do healthy things together. Before long, both men shared a house key but that was about all. Matt slipped into depression and isolation, refusing all help. He made impulsive financial decisions that robbed him of belongings and dignity, while increasing stress. He was mad at the world.

Matt met his niece, Devyn, as a newborn in the hospital. However, he was too focused on his deteriorating life circumstances and self-loathing to let her innocence and love penetrate. Superficially he knew the birth was cause for celebration, but he was numb to it. He needed to get unstuck before he could look up and step forward to seize the love that awaited him.

As Matt's personal life stabilized, fragile strands of family contact were reinforced through loving gestures of weekly contact and family dinners. The thick wax plug that sealed anger in and family out started to melt. Once the plug dissolved, the love for his biological niece began to flourish and thrive. An old soul in a young body, Devyn quietly but truly connected lovingly with her Uncle Matt. And then came baby number two—another niece, Alexandra Mae. She quickly earned the title *Alexandra Mayhem* for her antics, which always made Matt crack up. Known as Alex for short, she's a spitfire.

"So what shenanigans has Alex been up to today?" Matt would chuckle with tenderness in his voice. Initially he'd admonish Kate for not watching Alex closely enough until he got to spend more time with his young niece.

"She sure gets into things and moves super fast," he laughed when joining the family for Sunday dinner.

"Her mischievous smile and glowing eyes are the only hints that she is, or was, up to something," Kate responded as she nabbed and tickled a wiggly Alex. "I don't get much rest with this one."

"Oh, that sounds like Alex," Matt said. "But how'd she grab the margarine and leave those deep finger grooves without getting caught?"

"I think Kate blinked," was all I needed to say. Judgement of Kate had fallen to the wayside in equal proportion to the meteorological rise of love for his nieces.

151

By now our petite little Zoe rounded out the trio of sisters, all within a four-year span. Devyn adopted her big sister/mothering role with fervour and Alex was determined that she could do anything her big sister did. Devyn spilled knowledge and Alex was the paper towel that sopped it up. As for little Zoe, she quickly came into her own and earned the nickname, Alex 2.0. No wonder Matt gained a newfound respect and admiration for his sister.

Always eager to share his love of the transit system, Matt was proud when Kate gave permission to introduce Devyn to his passion, with me tagging along. Devyn was three and a half at the time. She and I waited at the bus shelter and later met Matt at the transit centre. We rode a bus, then the train, before walking to a playground. He was very attentive and Devyn enjoyed every moment, with the exception of a portion of the train ride, when it clanged and clattered through a pitch-black tunnel. Matt perceptively noted her nervousness.

When the time came to leave the playground and head home, he squatted to her level. "Devyn, was that scary going through the dark tunnel?" She bowed her head, casting her eyes downward.

With a gentle voice he said, "Uncle didn't mean to scare you. Would you like to go back home on the bus instead?" She eagerly nodded and squeezed his hand. "Okay let's have one last slide and then we'll go."

Once on the bus, Matt guided us to the long back row, which was a single step higher. From this vantage point he could oversee the whole bus. He gave Devyn the window seat for the best view. He sat next to her and I hemmed them in. Tired from the adventure, Devyn became lulled by the rhythm of the bus. I glanced over and saw her eyelids at half-mast and little hand stretched out on Uncle Matt's knee. Matt lovingly patted her hand. Feeling safe and secure, sleep beckoned. I smiled, relishing the healing of sibling relationships and forging new generational bonds.

The tranquility was broken when a dishevelled, unsteady man boarded the bus and sat in the back near us. He was wrapped in an invisible cape of mental health issues. Mumbling and grumbling turned into increasingly foul language, spewed at nobody in particular. Although words and demeanour didn't penetrate Devyn's consciousness, Matt and I were acutely aware of the man's growing agitation. Momentarily frozen, we neither spoke nor looked at each other. I weighed whether to risk saying something to this troubled man or approach the driver. Either way I needed to act soon.

Suddenly, "Hey, watch your language!" boomed from beside me.

Matt glared at the man, who scowled back. Matt didn't blink. I was prepared to intervene if the man became threatening, but hoped it could be avoided. The muttering quieted and the man rang the bell to get off at the next stop. He clearly didn't like our company. Nicely done, Uncle Matt!

Matt leaned over, saying "What a jerk! That was far beyond inappropriate. There's a little kid on this bus—and well, have to remember, you're a senior too." My turn to pat his knee.

Matt offered to babysit if Kate and Robby wanted an evening out. Kate appreciated the gesture but it was well beyond her comfort level. Matt's loving intentions and stress level could readily become overloaded by her dynamic trio and menagerie of pets. Then one evening—a surprise phone call.

"Matt, I have a favour to ask," Kate said. "I've been offered a cancellation spot at my doctor's in the morning. Robby's working. Would you be willing to watch the kids if I paid for cab fare and had oatmeal ready for all of you?"

The appointment was close to home. She'd be gone and back within an hour. A testing of the waters. Matt jumped at the chance and was giddy with exhilaration.

153

The next morning Matt arrived earlier than the scheduled time, to ensure Kate wouldn't be late. "Thanks, Matt. This really helps me out."

"No—thank you! I can't believe you're letting me do this. Hey Alex! You're such a little monkey-doodle! Give your Uncle Matt a big bear hug." She flew into his arms. "Good morning, Devyn. I like your pyjamas. Uncle needed to get out of his pyjamas early to come and babysit you." She laughed and ran away.

He picked up baby Zoe, kissed her and sniffed the air. "Is that oatmeal I'm smelling? Hope there's enough for me. Come on girls, Uncle Matt will get you some."

The babysitting went smoothly. He gave Kate a glowing report on how well behaved the girls were—pets too. Matt called that evening with his triumphant report.

"Mum, I called Robby when he finished work. After all, he is the father and I thought he should hear directly from me. We watched a Disney movie. Devyn and Alex curled up by me on the couch. Of course, Devyn told me silly jokes that made no sense. She laughed so hard at herself that she made me laugh too. Still don't know what was funny. I sure love those girls."

"Was Zoe sleeping?"

"Nope. She was with us. Instead of letting her sit on the floor I picked her up and put her on my knee. I wanted her to feel included as an important part of this family. I did a good job so hope to do it again someday."

"Maybe you will. I know Kate was pleased. Trusting you with her girls says a lot."

Matt was shocked when the following week Kate called upon him again. This time Kate and Zoe were headed away for the weekend. I was out of town and she needed to catch a cab to the airport before

154

rush hour. It would be about an hour before Robby would be home from work.

Matt called me later that evening. "So how was your babysitting gig?" I asked.

"Pretty good." He hesitated before continuing. "It's just that Alex got *hangry,* right after Kate left."

"Oh?"

"I tried to cuddle her but she didn't want to be touched. Then she shrieked and you know how much that hurts my ears."

"Sure do. For such a little girl, Alex has a high-pitched shrill."

"I asked her to stay calm but she didn't like that—guess 'cause she's only three. Knew I had to keep cool so she'd trust me and not be scared."

"So how did you handle it?"

"Went to the kitchen to find her something to eat. I gave her two arrowroot cookies and that helped. She calmed right down, so it worked out good."

"Glad to hear. And did you give any to Devyn?"

"Mum! Of course. I wouldn't leave her out. She got two so it would be fair. Robby came home a few minutes later."

"Did you give him a full report again?"

"No, just told him the girls were fine and then got a drive home. Didn't mention Alex yelling. Wanted her to know she can trust me, to not rat her out."

"Nice call, Matt. You're earning both their love and trust—important stuff."

Pride wafted into his voice. "True. I don't need any special title to be a truly great uncle."

Chapter 16: Game Day

My cousin Rose's comment came from left field, oh so long ago, in 1983. Bewildered, I remember asking, "So why might people think we named our baby after a football player?"

Chuckling on the phone, Rose said "Look at the cover of today's *Edmonton Journal* sports section. You'll see." She waited while I retrieved the newspaper.

There it was in bold print. The Edmonton Eskimos football team had just signed an American—Matt Dunigan. A record-breaking quarterback at the college level, "Dash" Dunigan was highly prized, yet considered too small for the National Football League. Given slim odds of American success, he opted for the Canadian Football League. His talents would be showcased with the Edmonton Eskimos, assuming the role of quarterback, since the legendary Warren Moon was retiring. After scanning the article, I returned to the phone.

"Omigod—I see what you mean! This new football star obviously isn't related as he spells his last name differently. There are a lot of Dunnigan's in Neil's clan and we chose our baby's name carefully. Neil checked with his aunt and uncle who had 12 children and 33 grandchildren, before settling on an unclaimed boy's name. Nobody could have predicted this. It'll be interesting to see how the tale of two Matts unfolds." I pinched myself to confirm I wasn't dreaming.

Matt Dunigan quarterbacked in Edmonton for five years, prior to playing for other CFL teams. Over the years he coached in Calgary, was inducted into the CFL Hall of Fame and became a veteran commentator at The Sports Network (TSN). Over that time, our family collected tales related to the namesake issue.

Our baby was only a few months old when Neil mentioned that he frequently saw football player Matt with his teammates at a favourite lunch spot. One day my husband spoke to the football player when both men were checking out the daily fare at the trattoria. Neil told adult Matt the namesake story and invited the young man to join us for a home-cooked dinner. Brand new to Edmonton, he expressed gratitude for the hospitality and an eagerness to meet baby Matt. A dinner date was set for that weekend.

On Saturday evening the assigned time came and went. We were about to give up when the embarrassed young man arrived over 45 minutes late. He apologized profusely, citing having lost track of time. Neil and I were quickly won over by his open, friendly and down-to-earth manner.

The football star scooped Matthew into his arms, held him out and with a very heavy Texan drawl said, "Well hello there Mattheeew, little budddy." Near the end of a relaxing dinner, he decided to elaborate on his late arrival and sparse appetite. Earlier that evening, after football practice, he couldn't shake a niggling feeling that he should be somewhere other than with his teammates. In the last few bites of his post-practice meal, he suddenly remembered our dinner engagement. Promptly leaving the restaurant, he rushed to our home, for a second hearty dinner. His stomach was pushed to the limit that night.

The two Matts met again years later when Matt Dunigan was coach of Calgary's CFL team and our young man was visiting a friend in Calgary. Our son heard that the Calgary Stampeders were practising at McMahon Stadium. He navigated his way there by bus. He asked to speak with the coach, citing their common name, initial meeting when he was a baby and topping off his plea by saying he was on a weekend visit from Edmonton. After waiting a few minutes our son's initiative was rewarded. He proudly told us about his accomplishment.

"Naturally I thanked him and showed him my ID. After all, I wanted him to know my visit was legit."

"What did you guys talk about, Matt?" I asked.

"We agreed that it was funny to have the same name and that we'd already met when I was a baby. Told him that even though he works for Edmonton's arch rival football team now, I still like him and am glad he's with the CFL. It was a good visit, but short 'cause he needed to get back to practice. Glad I dropped by."

"Good on you for taking the initiative—most other people would only have thought about doing it. That memory will always stay with you."

Matt puffed out his chest. "Definitely…and this time, I'm old enough to remember the meeting."

Over the years, when teaching his specialty course on non-abusive psychological and physical intervention across Alberta, Neil was routinely asked the same question. "Are you related to Matt Dunigan?"

Neil enjoyed seeing the mystified looks on participants' faces when he said, "Yes, I'm his father." Everyone knew the age gap wasn't that huge. Neil shared the namesake story and everyone got a good laugh.

Our Matt became an avid football fan. Post high school, Matt decided to invest in Edmonton Eskimos season tickets, as the franchise offered a payment plan. He was prepared to purchase his ticket with earnings from his part-time courtesy clerk job. Payment had to be paid in full before tickets were released, shortly before the season opener. This up-front instalment plan appealed to Matt, allowing him the opportunity to be a prestigious season ticket holder and plan his work schedule around home games.

"You know, Matt," I told him, "going with someone to a football game would be much more fun. So Dad and I are prepared to pay for a second set of tickets. That way you can always treat someone to a game—whoever you want."

"Cool! I'd like that. And don't worry, I'll take you guys too. I get paid on Friday, so can we go to the Esks office right after your work? I want to get the best seats I can afford and give my first down payment. You'll have your money ready, right?"

"Yes to all of the above. Going to one game will be enough for me—Dad too. Hard football seats are best suited for younger butts and backs."

Matt became a regular visitor at the Eskimos office, dropping in to pay his instalments and sometimes simply to say hello. An enthusiastic ambassador for the pending season, he developed an easy rapport with staff.

Matt hosted *nine* individuals to games throughout the season. Family, friends and colleagues all enjoyed the experience. Matt was particularly delighted when a guest sprung for hotdogs and a drink. He came home with tales of great touchdowns, bad calls, fireworks, overtime wins and losses, scorching sun and torrential downpours. It all added to a magical season of camaraderie and diverse experiences.

One lucky guest was a peer with significant disabilities. A lovely young man, Kyle lives with multiple layers of complexity. His unique challenges include being non-verbal and living with mobility issues. Garbled messaging between his brain and body often results in jerky, involuntary movements. Knowing Kyle would be thrilled to attend a game, Matt ran a proposed strategy by me.

"Mum you know how much I like buses. I want to take Kyle to the game by myself, on the bus. It'll mean a couple of transfers to get to his house and then to the game, but that's fine with me. Once at the Westmount Transit Centre we can catch the Game Day stadium bus. It's kinda cool on the bus 'cause everyone's excited. Lots wear Esks shirts, bring horns or have their faces painted green and gold. I bet Kyle would love it."

"I think so too. The Esks bus sounds like a party atmosphere. Kyle would be in his glory."

"But," Matt insisted, "there's no way I'd take him on the Game Day bus after the game. Lots of people who take that bus get really drunk at the game. I think 'cause they don't need to drive. Kyle has problems with balance so I wouldn't *ever* put him in danger of being knocked over on the ride back."

Then his tone shifted to the one he used when asking me for something. "Hoping you'll pick us up after the game and drive Kyle home. I promise parking won't be a problem 'cause we'd wait until most people leave. That avoids the risk of Kyle getting bumped in the crowd. Better to play it safe."

Matt's concern and attention to details spoke to how important this plan was to him. Considering all aspects of the evening required significant focus. His brain would have been on overdrive reviewing potential scenarios and risks. Ensuring his friend Kyle's safety was paramount.

"I like how well you've thought this through. And yes, I'm willing to do my part. So what's your next step to make this happen?"

"I'd need to call Kyle's parents and they can talk to him about the idea. Sure hope they say yes."

Matt wasted no time in asking for their phone number. All endorsed the plan and both young men eagerly awaited game day.

Matt left home hours before stadium doors opened, allowing ample time for bus connections to Kyle's house and their bus journey to the stadium. He stressed the importance of being safely settled in their steep seats before the venue got too busy. Matt promised to call me later when it was pickup time.

During the game, it was announced that the crowd's beloved former quarterback Matt Dunigan was on-site, providing game commentary for TSN. Naturally, our Matt decided it would be nice to reconnect and introduce his friend after the game. Waiting until the bleachers were almost empty, Matt and Kyle slowly wound their way down to the dressing rooms, in the bowels of the stadium. By the time they arrived, commentator Matt had left the building.

At least an hour later than the anticipated pickup time our phone rang. The dressing room detour had significantly delayed projected timelines.

"No need to worry, Mum." Oh how those words always put me on edge. "I know a shortcut to meet you at a perfect pickup spot. Meet you at the east side of the building in 10 minutes. Bye."

"No, no—Matt, don't hang up!" Luckily, he heard me. "I need an exact pickup location, to avoid driving round and round."

Pulling over by the designated flagpole, there was no exit gate in sight. In the distance, two animated lads made a beeline to the chain-link fence that separated the stadium grounds from the sidewalk. It was the most direct route from the dressing rooms to the road. Rolling down my window I overheard Matt encouraging Kyle to move faster. Kyle was doing his utmost to keep up, limbs flailing with laughter and excitement. I bore postgame witness to exuberant buddies, embracing their adventure—well worth the wait.

Their arrival at the fence provided fresh perspective. Like standing by a goal post, the barrier appeared much taller than when viewed from afar. The guys looked at the fence and each other. After huddling together, Matt stood back and clapped his hands. He'd devised a plan.

While standing at the base of this seemingly insurmountable hurdle, a police helicopter flew overhead. Being the early days of police helicopters in Edmonton, this rare sight captured the guys' attention. They looked at each other and in tandem sent obscene finger gestures skyward. The helicopter continued its flight path to an unknown destination.

Matt boosted Kyle, who struggled to climb the structure, while tugging on his pants. They were slipping dangerously low. This fumbled first attempt provided some learning. The pair needed to refine their strategy. Kyle's pants were firmly hiked up and Matt gave him a pep talk. I watched and waited in anticipation.

Like a quarterback determined to deliver, Matt dug deep and gave Kyle an extra boost, straining to keep his friend inching closer to the goal line. With Kyle teetering near the top, Matt grunted and gave a final push. Time was suspended as Kyle's butt kissed and bounced along the grass strip that bordered the sidewalk. A hard-earned touchdown!

Learning from Kyle's ascent, Matt managed to scale the fence in one attempt. Matt opened the rear passenger door for his friend and helped him buckle the seatbelt. Turning to Kyle I asked if he had fun. He gave me two thumbs up. That's when I noticed he was unbalanced.

"Oh no Kyle, you've only got one shoe on! Where's the other?" Kyle looked down at his sock foot, slapped his forehead with his hand and broke into hysterical laughter. "Matt, help me out here," I blurted.

"Mum, I know he had two shoes on." Turning to Kyle, Matt said, "Must've come off when you went over the fence, pal." Matt ran from the car and peered through the chain-link fence, his face pressed against the cool metal. The night sky was rapidly laying down a blanket of darkness.

"See it! Yup, right where he tried climbing the first time. I'll get it for ya, Kyle." I was mesmerized by Matt's rare bout of agility as he focused on retrieving his friend's lost apparel. Like his namesake, at that moment in time he could rightly be called "Dash" Dunnigan.

Waving the prized possession in the air, Matt opened the rear passenger door. He and Kyle exchanged high fives. "Kyle, my man, I'll help you get your shoe on—just stick your foot out for me. Can't quite believe that you lost it—or even better, that I found it!"

Kyle whooped with laughter and it became contagious. The car was a cacophony of hoots, howls, snorts and thigh slapping. It took a few minutes before my vision cleared enough to drive. I felt like a chauffeur driving these raucous buddies home after a triumphant night on the town.

A decisive win for the home team!

Chapter 17: The Ask

I'd repeatedly scoured every recess of my mind, to no avail. Hope was waning fast. Then a ludicrous fantasy floated by when I saw him in the cereal aisle. Did I have the nerve to act? By the weekend I summoned the courage to ask.

The request was both simple and incredibly complex. The risk required one phone call and full exposure. Damn that one potentially insurmountable hurdle. All other bases were covered— vacation time, creative budget crunching, dedication to training, and cherished travelling companions. The near certainty of being left behind had me teetering on the precipice of despair and resentment.

Shoulders hugged my ears and I stared at my kitchen phone. One massive stress ball, my sweaty fist released the crumpled paper with his phone number. It was his day off and I had a rare hour home alone. The perfect time, perhaps the only time.

My mouth was dry, heart racing, hands trembling. After many false starts, I picked up the phone and dialled John. It rang and panic set in. "Please pick up; no, no please don't. What if his wife answers?"

"Hello?" I took a deep, calming breath. This was uncharted territory, fraught with guilt and fear. I needed to slay this dragon with one fell swoop. "Hi John, it's Susan, Matt's mother. Hope you can spare a minute—have something outrageous to ask."

We first met John when Matt was little, during a routine grocery shop. These expeditions were like being thrust into a game of Russian Roulette; tension was my constant companion, regardless of duration. Matt always scampered ahead, eager to see what treasures the next aisle held. It was a good omen when I heard him announce, "Knew it—look who's stocking shelves!" John looked down on Matt with those sparkling hazel eyes and asked: "Find any good bargains yet today? Mum okay with you having a treat?" He reached for a candy in his blue apron pocket.

I knew John superficially at best. Never had coffee with him, nor met his wife and didn't know if he owned a dog. Just knew that I always trust my gut and for this request, John was my man. Reminiscent of the Catholic confessional of my youth, I blurted out my sinful desires. With this heavy burden lifted I took a much-needed breath.

Pausing momentarily, John said, "Well I'd need to check my work schedule and talk with my wife, Penny."

"Yes, yes of course! No pressure, really, I'd just need to know within the next couple of weeks." And that's where we left it.

The phone call had ignited a small glimmer of hope—fragile yet vital. Needing to share my elation, I called my friend and colleague Leigh. She understood the multilayered complexities of my life.

"Omigod Leigh, I've asked somebody I barely know if Matt could live with his family for two weeks, while I travel halfway around the globe for karate training. Hard to believe he didn't turn me down flat! It sounds like he might actually consider it."

"Wow, Susan! Can't imagine the courage it…"

"Must admit it was nerve-racking. Somehow managed to get my words out without breaking down. And to be truthful, if I can't go…." I dug my fingernails into my hands, and then decided to trust Leigh with my emotions. "Well, I'd cry to and from the airport. Some black belt colleagues are taking their wives along, as a vacation. It's not fair that despite training for decades I might get left behind. God, I'm already brewing a concoction of resentment and guilt, even though it's nobody's fault. Working full time, managing the karate school in Neil's absence and keeping the peace at home could take me over the edge."

166

When I shakily drew an overdue deep breath, Leigh seized the moment. "Oh, Susan, I marvel at how you relentlessly juggle challenges. Working in the field of disability and living it 24/7 are worlds apart. Somehow you manage to stay firmly rooted in both realms."

"I advocate as best I can, while understanding system and personal realities. Feeling worn out though and need a break to regroup."

"Understandably. Work's relentless and Matt presents as such an enigma. On one hand he is bright and capable, which raises expectations." Leigh's understanding felt like being wrapped in a warm blanket.

"Yes indeed. All too often his struggles to process common logic, risks and consequences get easily dismissed as an oddity, not a disability. And then well-intentioned people offer simple solutions to this complex puzzle. Walk a mile...."

Matt, who had recently turned 22, was adamant that he could manage independently for two weeks, even with his dad and me in Okinawa. "Just trust me and go, Mum. I can handle it and keep a good eye on my pesky sister too." Kate rolled her eyes and returned to buttering a sandwich.

"Now Kate, if Mum goes, I won't stand for you inviting rowdy friends over for beer around the firepit."

She put the knife down. "You're such a jerk, Matt! I'm almost 18, not 12! I'd never do such a stupid thing. Can't you *ever* just leave me alone?" Kate walked out in a huff. I glared at Matt.

"Why are you giving me a dirty look? Those kinds of things can happen, you know. I'm the older brother and won't put up with any of her shenanigans."

Forever a fine balancing act—supporting Matt discreetly and respectfully, while ensuring proper safeguards and minimizing

167

clashes with his younger sister. At 17, Kate was very responsible and routinely stayed at her best friend's on weekends. Those sleepovers provided a refuge from the constant reprimands of her brother.

Transforming the trip from dream to reality required Matt being supported by someone our whole family respected and whose oversight buffered Kate from her domineering brother. Kate always had the option of staying at a friend's if sibling tensions got too high during weekdays. Backup plans have always been as important as the primary plan.

I saw John a few times when shopping during the next two weeks. He said nothing and I was too afraid to ask. Every minute dragged its heavy weight over me. Nights were broken by interrupted sleep and recurring dreams of rejection. Tension and worry tightened their screws.

Every day, I checked seat availability for the flight my husband and friends booked. Numbers steadily dwindled. Then one day—a single seat left! Feet barely touching the floor, I grabbed the phone, bracing myself for the letdown.

John's response casually rolled off his tongue. "Penny and I've talked about it. She wonders if Matt might be more comfortable staying at home, with me visiting daily, working around my schedule."

"Wow, um, I can't quite believe what I'm hearing. Penny is obviously a generous woman, with a good heart and even better instincts. Having Matt stay at home respects his dignity as a man. It'll consume a lot of time and energy on your part, so think about what you'd like for compensation."

"Well, there's definitely no need for any payment. Matt tells me he likes to cook. He can show me his culinary skills and we'll have fun while we're at it."

"That's extremely magnanimous." Hesitatingly I dared to add, "You do remember this trip is for two full weeks, right?"

"Sure do. That's not a problem. It's a good opportunity to get to know my friend Matt better."

Alone in the house, my jubilation bounced off the walls, "Yahoo—I'm going to Okinawa!"

Matt was receptive—pleased even—with this opportunity to show his friend and former colleague how responsible and capable he was at home. John's diligence and oversight allowed Neil and me to embrace Okinawan culture, friendship and karate training.

Ironically during our trip Matt's own actions triggered his anxiety about raucous parties. A few weeks before the trip, two buddies had invited Matt to join them for Saturday night revelry at a bar. Late the next morning, Matt beamed when he entered the kitchen.

"Well that turned out to be a surprisingly successful night. The place was jam-packed and too loud to even talk—got boring, fast. So I found the manager and asked if they needed help clearing tables. And he offered me a job, starting right away. I made enough money to catch a cab home and even stopped at a 7-Eleven for a pop."

"Oh Matt," I groaned. Images of him trying to intervene in bar fights and bottles whizzing through the air populated every brain cell. The timing of this latest job was far from good. Life carried on and we embarked on our trip.

As planned, Kate spent the weekend at her friend's. Matt was working at the bar on Saturday night. Impulsiveness got the best of him as his shift drew to a close. Anxious about going home to an empty house, he posted an invitation in the men's washroom, providing our home address. Cocooned in the sanctuary of the bus heading home, Matt watched Saturday night partiers spill into the streets. That's when actions and potential consequences connected in his brain. It was too late to remove the sign at the bar so he did the next best thing. Matt raced home, ensuring all doors and windows were locked. Then he made the midnight call.

John sprang into action. He put the police on alert and went to support Matt. John and Penny stayed until nearly 3 o'clock. Knowing his sleep would soon be disrupted again at 5:30, John could only doze. Dawn brought another workday.

Matt intended to heed John's advice to go to bed, but the adrenaline still sprinted in his veins. Using *Matt logic*, he opted for some fresh air in the park behind our house. Maybe telling his sister about his mistake might help him relax more. Taking the cordless phone with him he made his next call, staying within range of the house.

"Kate...you awake?"

"Not until now. It's after 3 a.m. so this better be important. What's up?"

Quickly gathering her wits, she listened incredulously, convinced him to take some deep breaths, and then head back inside to bed. She stayed on the phone until he was safely home. The reassuring sound of the deadbolt was swiftly followed by "Kate, I can't talk anymore; I'm too tired. Night."

Reassuring her bewildered friend with, "Matt's just being Matt," she returned to sleep.

After our return from Okinawa, we invited John and Penny over for a post-trip thank-you dinner. It was the least we could do to thank them for opening their hearts and being so responsive.

During dinner Penny turned to me and said, "Did you know that we support my brother who also lives with an intellectual disability?"

"No, I had no idea. That's likely why intuitively I knew to ask John. It explains your infinite wisdom and sensitivity, even though you'd never met Matt. You both have new insights now." We all laughed.

170

"Susan, you told me everything I needed to know about supporting Matt. Still," John confessed, "it quickly became clear that I only absorbed that information at a superficial level. Proof that experience is the best teacher."

"Like my simple, yet bold ask, things typically run deeper than they appear on the surface."

John raised his wine glass, proposing a toast, "To friendship and deeper understanding...."

Locking eyes, I added, "And let's not forget courage—the key that opens doors of possibility."

Chapter 18: Heartfelt

Life is a colourful explosion of tastes and textures. Tantalizing bite-size samples offer delicacies and scraps worth exploring, or avoiding. A penchant for sweet, salty or spicy depends on the individual palate. What one person devours another spits out. But without sampling, we never know. We tear, chew and swallow morsels of life that sometimes appear in unanticipated and improbable situations.

A memorable Saturday at the farmers' market was one such occasion. When scanning for a lunch table, I abruptly stopped. My heart skipped a beat.

"Follow me, hon—just spotted the perfect tablemates."

Feet skimming the ground, I bobbed and weaved through the crowd before arriving at the desired destination. Neil looked perplexed that I'd walked past closer options.

The duo, a father-daughter combo, kindly agreed to shimmy down, so we could join them. Sharing wooden picnic tables at the farmers' market was commonplace. Focused on his hotdog, not our tablemates, I tapped Neil's shin with my foot. My eyes glanced towards the slight teenage girl who sat beside him enjoying her lunch. Neil's raised eyebrows assured me the unspoken message was received. Time to probe.

Wiping hotdog mustard from the corner of my mouth I introduced us, deliberately offering first and last names. The girl's father responded in kind. A fact-finding mission, under the guise of casual conversation. By the time we parted ways I knew where he worked, reaffirmed initial impressions and got the sense that disability-related connections weren't on this family's radar.

On Monday morning, my vague message at the man's place of work requested a call, as a "follow-up to an earlier conversation." I hoped curiosity and my government phone number might prompt a response. Maybe this would lead somewhere, or nowhere at all. Larry called later that day.

I began. "This call will probably sound strange, but let me explain. It stems from sharing a lunch table on Saturday. Both my husband and I were struck by your daughter's traits, which are remarkably similar to our son's. We wondered if you might be interested in hearing what caught our attention." He was.

We talked about physical features and a propensity to be socially precocious—characteristics our teenagers shared. With Larry's permission I dove a bit deeper, exploring other similarities. He became totally engaged when asked if Lily had extreme noise sensitivity, anxiety and early childhood developmental delays. His eagerness to know more was palpable.

"Susan, everything you've raised is bang on. It's like you know Lily intimately. Actually, it's…it's quite overwhelming." It struck me that I'd used almost the same phrasing years before.

"Larry, the common traits I've raised are based solely on observations over hotdogs and parental experiences raising a child diagnosed with Williams Syndrome. That's the extent of my expertise. To explore this further I'd suggest you talk with your doctor and request a consultation with the genetics clinic. A genetic consultation is how we got Matt's diagnosis. Good luck, and thanks for being curious enough to call. I'll give you my home number, in case you ever want to talk again." Months went by.

One Saturday morning Matt answered the phone. "Yes, this is Matthew. My mum? She's right here doing the dishes, but sure she won't mind stopping." He handed me the phone whispering, "It's a man. He sounds very nice."

"Susan, it's Larry. I followed your suggestion and wanted to share how it went. After a lot of persuasion from my wife and me, our doctor referred us to the genetics clinic. The wait seemed eternal—but that's all behind us now." His voice revealed a hairline fracture. "We have a diagnosis … Williams Syndrome." I heard him swallow.

"Larry, any chance you and your family would like to drop by for coffee and a visit? We're home all day today or tomorrow." Our doorbell rang mid-afternoon.

Lily and Matt exchanged polite introductions before launching into stream-of-consciousness chatter, as if long lost friends. Both sets of parents marvelled at the ease of this peer-to-peer connection. Unique traits that typically made our kids stand out as "different" faded away. Families immediately connected by a common bond.

Lily joined Matt when he went to the kitchen for a plate of cookies. Kate's neutral face softened having witnessed Lily's nervous glance at the ceiling's smoke detector, when passing through the hallway. We exchanged a knowing mother-daughter glance.

Matt offered to show Lily the house, which she promptly accepted. His tour was thorough—back entry, bathroom, litter box corner and basement included. Upstairs was next. From the living room we overheard Matt's cautious voice.

"Lily, hold the banister really tight. These stairs are steep and you're not wearing slippers. If you want, I can take your hand at the landing, 'cause there's no railing there. Ready?"

An excited Lily announced their return. "Whoa, Matt's room is amazing! It's like being at a movie theatre, with posters covering every wall. Even complete with bits of popcorn on the floor." Turning to her parents she added, "Don't worry, I stepped over it, not in it."

Matthew slapped his forehead and blushed. "Oops! Obviously missed some in my rush to clean up. Think I made up for the mess by letting you choose some spare posters. Remember you were going to ask your parents if you can go with me to a matinee next Saturday." Before Lily could say a word, he addressed her parents. "It's all part of being a Paramount employee. I get free admission and can take a guest, anytime."

As we wrapped up the visit, Kate returned plates and cups to the kitchen. Lily followed, carrying the cream and sugar bowls. Kate went through the dining room, which avoided the hallway smoke detector.

"Kate, I'm so glad my parents said yes to the movies with Matt next week. Your brother is soooo nice."

"I'm glad you got along so well. I usually don't go to movies with him, but love the leftover concession stand popcorn he brings home. On weekdays I take it for a recess snack—makes my friends jealous."

"Kate, you are so lucky to have him."

"Maybe…doesn't usually feel that way. Do you and your brother always get along?"

"Definitely not. Probably like that with all brothers." Both girls laughed and Lily spontaneously hugged Kate goodbye.

The next Saturday, Lily's parents dropped her off at our home. I was the designated chauffeur to and from the theatre. Matt had a bus pass so didn't usually get a ride, but Lily wasn't as independent. Waiting for Lily's parents to pick her up, the pair rehashed movie highlights. The successful movie venture paved the way for another the following week.

Lily was totally smitten and called daily. Her emotional exuberance highlighted another shared trait, the emotional "10-times factor." Matt stood taller after each call, clinging to every word that stroked his ego. This was the first time he'd been the recipient of romantic attention.

Two items of childhood memorabilia hinted at early romantic yearnings. In an elementary-school note Matt asked to share slow dances at the school dance, if it was okay with the girl's boyfriend, Matt's buddy. In junior high he invited a girl to the graduation dance. The teen wrote a sweet note back, saying she was flattered

175

but needed to decline. The girl was going with another classmate, her boyfriend.

Lily awaited her parents' arrival gazing out the living room window after the second matinee. Deep in thought she startled when Kate walked into the room.

"Sorry Kate—didn't mean to jump. Funny, just thinking about you. Matt's gone to his bedroom looking for Scooter. Need to give that sweet cat a goodbye rub." Lily looked towards the stairs and lowered her voice. "I've been thinking and have a question I'd like to ask you. Your timing's perfect."

"Don't worry. The stairs always creak on the way down, so that'll be our warning. What's up?"

"Well we've seen two movies now and your brother is my knight in shining armour. I'm wondering, if Matt and I ever decide to get married someday, would you be my maid of honour? It would mean the world to me." With fists clenched against her chest in anticipation, Lily stared eagerly into the depth of Kate's full-moon eyes.

After a moment of recovery, Kate's words tumbled out. "I'm glad you like my brother so much. Most girls dream about getting married someday. Of course, I'd have no say in Matt getting married or not. But, if you ever became his bride, I'd gladly be your maid of honour. But no rushing it, okay?"

The stairs squeaked and a vibrating Lily nodded that she understood. For the next few minutes Lily cuddled Scooter and looked lovingly at Matt. Then her parents pulled up to the curb and she said her goodbyes.

As soon as the front door closed Kate called, "Mum, where are you? Need to talk—holy crap!"

Our daughter's empathetic and sensitive nature was evident to all, except maybe her brother. This was the first time I caught a glimpse of her quick-witted diplomatic skills. Well done, my girl!

Matt and Lily's Saturday outings expanded beyond movie matinees, to include lunches and coffee dates with Matt's cousin Martin and his wife. Matt proudly gave Lily a nickname, adopting the exact one that Martin called his spouse. Lily was thrilled. Their dating started when Matt was 17 and lasted three years. The relationship endured beyond graduation from high school and his college program.

As with all relationships, the initial shine dulled, expectations changed and other interests emerged. Moving away and living in a college dorm, Matt experienced freedom away from the watchful eyes of parents. He experimented with the scope of what young adulthood had to offer. It was during his turbulent college days that Matt sustained a traumatic head injury. After college, Lily was elated to have him home, as evidenced by the multiple daily phone calls.

"Lily, stop calling so much! Jeez, just talked with you an hour ago," Matt grumbled. Then holding the kitchen phone far from his ear, he exhaled a loud exasperated sigh. Neil's eyes chastised Matt's tone and actions. Matt returned the phone to his ear, listened for a moment and then responded contritely.

"Lily, I care about you too. But really there's nothing new to talk about—just that I'm eating lunch. Don't like making you upset, but so many calls are driving me totally bonkers. Please try to call just once a day, like we've talked about—lots."

Relationship tension and instability mounted. Anxious, scared and unsure of her footing, Lily clung tighter. Matt's resentment and impatience flared. Feeling smothered and with a short fuse, the explosion was only a matter of time. Matt's appetite for overwhelming sweetness was gone. He'd had his fill, so unceremoniously spit it out. When he yelled at Lily to get out of his life, he meant it. Devastated, she did.

Oh, how many times I'd snapped at Matt, in a similar vein, when caught in the vortex of his anxiety, perseverance and heightened emotions. My angry words begged for a reprieve—just a few minutes or hours. Regardless of duration, the underlying message screamed annoyance and dismissal. Sometimes Matt walked away with slumped shoulders, leaving me teetering between shame and survival. My every cry for personal space inadvertently contributed drip by drip to cumulative societal messages that filled his soul with a sense of unworthiness. Judged as different—and not in a good way.

Without Lily there was a hole in Matt's life. A welcome break initially, he eagerly accepted a college buddy's invitations to go out, often to bars. Loud music and superficiality bombarded all captives, masquerading as a good time. Matt wanted to fit in, but didn't meet the cool threshold. His flamboyant friend brimmed with confidence, propped up by ample cash, trendy clothes, flashy bling...and a car. Matt was a tag-along, physically deep in the bowels of party central, yet emotionally outside looking in.

Although Matt didn't regret the break-up with Lily, shame haunted him for the hurt inflicted by his angry dismissal. He and this sweet young woman were much alike in regards to diagnostic traits, but miles apart on other fronts. Healthy female attention continued to elude him.

One day after a shopping expedition, two young women spotted Matt at the bus stop, where he was repacking groceries on the bench. He'd inadvertently pulled the cord early, hopping off the bus a stop too soon. Preoccupied with redistributing bag weight for his walk home, they initiated contact.

"Hey bud, can we help?"

"Huh? Oh, no thanks. Guy did a lousy job packing my groceries. He obviously didn't get good training, like when I worked at Safeway. Have to walk three blocks, so adjusting my load."

"Oh steaks! They sure look delicious. Haven't had a juicy steak in a long time," one of the young women said. Her companion agreed.

Matt smiled. "Couldn't pass up the great deal—it's buy one get one free this week."

"Just like us," one tittered.

"Had dinner yet? Don't live far away. Treating myself to steak and have enough to share. Want to come over?"

"Always appreciate good meat." Stifling smirks they added, "We'd love to come."

"Then let's go. Would you mind carrying a bag each since I'm loaded down?"

"No problem. Happy to lighten your load—just give me a second," said one young woman. After a hushed phone call, she picked up a grocery bag and they headed to his apartment. Shiny bait sent to lure in dinner.

Safely inside our son's apartment, their real motives surfaced. When Matt told them to leave, one snatched his keys. The other called their handler who she'd alerted earlier, and was waiting outside. She buzzed him up. Once apartment keys were passed to their boss, the women dutifully went in search of another target. The smoothly executed shakedown was routine for the trio, but terrifying for Matt.

The intimidating intruder insisted they drive to the nearest ATM for Matt to withdraw cash, in return for his apartment keys. Steering the man away from a closer option, Matt wisely identified the neighbourhood 7-Eleven as their destination. Familiar with the layout, Matt obediently walked towards the ATM, bankcard in hand, then dashed into the bathroom and locked the door. Grabbing the cell phone in his pocket, he called.

I excused myself from karate class to answer the phone. The panicked whisper sent chills up my spine.

"Come quick! Locked myself in the 7-Eleven washroom. Guy outside wants money before he'll give back my keys."

"What? Forget details—you're scaring me. Stay locked in the bathroom. I'll change and be there within five minutes."

With a pale face and pounding heart, I disrupted class, breathlessly sharing with Neil. "No context, but need to act. You keep teaching class. If anything goes sideways, I won't hesitate to call 911. Expect an update soon."

"Susan, be careful. I'd respond faster than 911 and be there in a flash." Feeling Neil beside me in spirit, I bolted.

Pulling on my boots to leave, two classmates unexpectedly appeared behind me. Conflicted, Neil shared his angst with these friends. Without a spoken word, Tony and John immediately bowed out of class. They already had coats on.

"Got your back, Susan. Won't let anyone hurt Matt."

"Gotta love you guys! See you there." I raced to my car.

At the 7-Eleven, I made a beeline for the washroom, noting a man lurking at the nearby magazine rack. John arrived moments later and was in lockstep behind me.

Catching sight of us the man hurriedly left the store to unlock his car. Parked nearby, Tony stepped out of his vehicle, made eye contact with the shakedown artist and wouldn't look away. A message was delivered—our son had people who looked out for him. The intended catch slipped off the hook. The man sped away, but not before rolling down his window and tossing Matt's keychain deep into the parking lot's dumpster.

After leaving our fearless friends, I used my spare key to secure Matt's apartment, grab his pyjamas, and then drive us home for the night. Our family debrief occurred sitting around the kitchen table. Matt was both rattled by the incident and upset with himself.

"Stupidhead me! Thought those girls were just being friendly, so offered to share a good dinner. Turned out to be a dirty trick." His embarrassment weighed heavy on my heart.

"Main thing is you're safe with your dad and me now. Those girls are expected to be super friendly to strangers—it's part of their job—a nasty, dangerous job. In their own way, they're trapped in scary situations, just like you were."

"I guess. Still a dirty trick, but the trick was on them—only had a few dollars left in my account so the ATM wouldn't have spit out money. That scary jerk probably wouldn't have given my keys back either way."

Putting his hand on our son's shoulder Neil said, "Don't beat yourself up too much. You ran into a team of pros who take advantage of people." Capitalizing on Matt's attentiveness he continued. "Friendly is good, but when strangers are overly friendly that should set off alarm bells in your head. Those girls reeled you in and backed it up by muscle. It scared all of us and put you in harm's way. Be proud that you got out of a risky situation by using your head. Guaranteed, we'll install a new door lock at your place tomorrow. Until then, get some sleep."

Drooping self-esteem pulled Matt into a deep sinkhole. Quality of life unravelled thread by thread. No relationship, personal or professional, was exempt from Matt's rage at the unfairness of it all. Isolation became his closest companion. His heart became frozen, sealed in dormancy, until an ember ignited from within.

Healed sibling wounds and a loving role as Uncle Matt stoked this ember. With a rekindled spirit Matt began to relinquish hefty boots of shame and self-loathing.

"Mum, I'm ready to get more people back in my life, so I'm not lonely. I want to get more active in the community and have stuff to do. Finding a part-time job would probably help and give me spending money too."

181

"You bet! Friends, community involvement and paid work help everyone feel valued and not so alone. So think about what steps you'd like to explore. The ball's in your court."

Life never guarantees meaningful relationships, romantic or otherwise, and it gives no refunds for mismatches. Although never stingy, life can sting for all citizens—sometimes enticing with the sweetness of honey. It's spectrum of sweet, sour and stickiness brings us wisdom and sometimes love. Matt simply wants his rightful share.

Section 2· Embracing Citizenship

Chapter 19: Emancipation Inc.

Flyers stuffed every mailbox along our street. Bright green notices with black typeface were designed to catch homeowners' attention and provide detailed information.

THE LAWN BOY, Serving People Since 1993 was the header. Bullet points cited key lawnmower features and the full range of services available. The flyer ended with a footnote, "Seniors get 35% off—all the time."

Our 10-year-old looked down the street, admiring every speck of green that poked from mailboxes. "Definitely chose the best colour 'cause it's the same as grass."

Business was brisk so he invited his best friend and close neighbour Gary to be his partner. They worked hard, laughed often and ended workdays with cold Slurpees from the 7-Eleven. The partnership lasted until Gary became a teen and was recruited to help out in his family's trucking business. Although paths diverged, the friendship remained, as did Matthew's insatiable quest for knowledge and connections.

Young Matthew exuded confidence and was eager to prove himself. He had no qualms about approaching the "boss of the vegetables" or sharing observations at the customer service desk.

"Matthew, let me know if you'd like any help from me."

"Jeez, Mum. I am capable. Wait over there. I'll wave if I need you." With routine practice, we got our respective roles down pat.

Quality customer service has always been paramount to Matthew, whether on the giving or receiving end. Approaching a store clerk, Matt introduced himself, asked their name and then launched into the issue at hand. Promotional queries, defective purchases, risks he noticed during our shopping expedition—it was all part of Matt's territory as far as he was concerned. I waited within earshot,

184

prepared to jump in if needed. My cue was his standard phrase "And my mum will tell you the rest."

Only when summoned could I provide more clarity or details. Sometimes my call came early. At other times it was later during the exchange. Matthew was proudest when he didn't need to call me at all. Those exchanges usually ended with Matt and the clerk exchanging friendly goodbyes and, "see you again soon."

Body language conveyed surprise at Matthew's exuberance, politeness, vocabulary and directness. He always found a way to connect on a personal level, commenting on whatever he appreciated about the person and the service he received. It was commonplace for grumpy-faced staff to soften their features, lose the frown and adopt a hint of a smile over the course of the discussion. Matt's enthusiasm and adventuresome spirit encouraged me to push boundaries.

A brochure about the first national Williams Syndrome conference in Toronto caught my attention. Youth sessions were available for those aged 15 or older. Despite Matthew being only 13, I made a case for him joining me. He became the youngest participant. The conference experience offered us new ideas, knowledge and a broader social network—all relevant to Life in the Matt Lane. Everything about the trip excited him—the flight from Edmonton, staying in a hotel, attending youth sessions and taking advantage of Toronto attractions—all within the confines of a three-day conference.

Arriving late at night, he marvelled at the lights of the big city from our 12th-floor hotel room. Bouncing up and down he pointed at the night sky.

"Look, Mum…I see it! Wow, the CN Tower—need to go there for sure. Hockey Hall of Fame too. And…"

"First things first—it's bedtime. Sessions start early in the morning. We'll take in as many sights as possible. Conference schedule looks busy though."

"Omigod, this place has a pool too. We definitely need to go swimming." With one hand on my hip, I yawned and pointed to his bed.

Early the next morning, he repeatedly pushed the elevator button while tightly pressing a conference folder against his chest. When the doors opened, the elevator was crammed with other guests eager to get their days started.

Matthew boldly stepped in, where no obvious space existed. I wasn't about to be left behind. To accommodate, strangers nestled uncomfortably close—sardines in a can. Shoulder to shoulder, we faced everyone, without a smidgen of space to turn around. The woman who I pressed up against had lipstick on a tooth, but I wasn't about to point it out. Only Matthew was oblivious to the awkwardness. Then he broke the code of elevator silence.

"Morning everyone. Thanks for squishing us in—goin' to my first conference." His smile went from ear to ear and a few faces brightened. "First time in Toronto too—sure have lots of fun things planned." A voice from the back said, "Wish I had fun things planned—nothing but boring meetings for me." People snickered and I relaxed.

Whenever the elevator stopped at a floor, Matthew swivelled his head as the door opened. "Sorry, too full. Good luck with the next one!"

Like a game of tag Matthew's joyful smile passed from person to person. At one floor a teenager and parent held conference folders too. "Hope the next one has room. Don't worry, I'll find you at the conference—my name is Matthew." Then the doors shut.

When we arrived at the main lobby, some patrons lingered briefly, connecting with Matthew. My son received well wishes as well as

186

general directions for the CN Tower and the nearest subway station. "Well those sure were nice people."

Agreeing, I looked up and noticed that the departing throng all seemed to have a spring in their step. The encounter with Mr. Enthusiasm started their day off on a positive note.

Matthew unreservedly embraced the sessions for youth, while I sopped up learning from the parental sessions. Following his lead, we made the most of every hour, squeezing in major sights. Matthew insisted on trying the subway he'd heard about. We ventured aboard, going uncomfortably far afield. Doors opened and without warning Matthew stepped off onto the platform and waved for me to join him. I needed to wrestle back control.

"Enough. It's getting late and we need to find out where our hotel is before taking another step." We'd travelled in so many directions while sightseeing that I was totally lost. Why hadn't I brought a map?

Matthew slowly and deliberately scanned the terrain, encompassing a full circle, one way, then the other. His second turn had confirmed something recognizable in the distance. Like a bloodhound, he was on the scent.

"Just trust me, Mum. We have to walk really fast to get back on time. Don't want to miss the big dinner and dance."

His good instincts rewarded us. Prolonged power-walking and vaguely familiar landmarks guided us. Exhausted, we arrived at the hotel, dropped our coats and hustled to the ballroom.

"Good timing, Mum—most people are eating so the food line-up's short. Hurry, I'm super hungry."

Lights dimmed, music started, and the dance floor swarmed with people. Not interested in dancing, Matthew approached the stage, the epicentre of activity. The welcoming DJ plopped his hat on Matthew's head and appointed him assistant for the evening. I relaxed and enjoyed the company of other families for a few hours. Stifling yawns, I turned to the stage. The DJ had his hat on, and my son was nowhere in sight. Reassuring myself and taking slow deep breaths, I applied *Matt logic*. I found him standing outside the hotel's locked swimming pool—checking out the hours of operation.

"Good tracking, Mum. Must be learning from me. Past bedtime now but let's still get up at 6 a.m. so we can swim before breakfast and packing. Good idea, hey?" One of many memorable adventures with Mr. Ingenuity.

Era Rowles, Matthew's former elementary-school teacher, believed in Matthew's capacity, both in and outside of school. She has retained an important role in his life, ebbing and flowing into adulthood. Eager to develop skills as a businessman, one summer, at about age 15, Matthew spent a lot of time at Rowles & Company Art Gallery. He considered it an unofficial apprenticeship. Era taught him to meticulously wrap gifts despite his dexterity issues, meeting her high standards and far exceeding my skill. He was introduced to the range of activities that filled Era's busy days.

She knew the importance of clear boundaries and employed strategies to challenge Matthew in positive ways. The only rub was consistently balking at taking direction from anyone assigned with authority, during Era's absence. His refrain, "She's not the boss of me," had a familiar ring to it.

One day Matthew came home pumped with excitement. Era had extended a highly prized opportunity. "Mum, I need to wear dress pants and a nice shirt 'cause I'm going with Era into lawyers' offices and places like that. She's delivering art and some pieces are too big for her. She trusts me to help her get it there safely. I take that very seriously. Think I need a tie?"

"That's quite an honour. Definitely want to look professional. Don't think a tie's needed though. Let's check your closet and choose something appropriate."

Helping Era with deliveries became routine that summer. Her customers shared how much they enjoyed meeting our son, who now preferred being called Matt. He proudly introduced himself as Era's assistant, often commenting on their good taste in artwork. On her solo trips, customers often inquired about Era's exuberant assistant.

One day, Matt and I were a few minutes early for a specialist's appointment. He wandered around the well-appointed waiting room, closely examining the artwork on the walls. After a few minutes of close scrutiny, I caught his eye and patted the chair beside me. Returning to his chair, Matt shook his head and seemed baffled.

"What's up?"

"I'm just surprised. Not a single piece of artwork is original—no limited-edition prints or even good reproductions. See how good I'm getting at recognizing quality? Maybe I'll mention Era's gallery to the doctor." His voice filled the quiet space. I put my index finger to my pursed lips, shaking my head.

The receptionist's bowed head lifted from her paperwork. She peered over her glasses, seemingly amused by Matt's observation. I feigned reading an article, until a nurse called us into the doctor's office.

As I walked past the receptionist, she straightened up and crooked her finger to come hither. With a twinkle in her eye she whispered, "I've always said the office art budget was beyond skimpy. Sounds like your son agrees."

Matt's unpaid apprenticeship as a young teen was educational, fulfilling and a stepping stone to paid employment. His first paid job, at age 16, was arranged through the AACL. They matched his love of movies with an employer who believed in supporting inclusion. Matt's work at the Paramount Theatre offered peer assistance until such time as he was comfortable and skilled enough to work independently. For Matt that support only lasted two shifts. His refrain of "I am capable" was fully endorsed by the assigned peer support. She was quickly reassigned to somebody else in need.

Matt loved his job, which started off with greeting guests, taking tickets and cleaning the theatre. He saw every aspect of his work as a component of good customer service. After each evening shift, he came home with at least one huge bag of leftover popcorn. We devoured what we could and my colleagues enjoyed any surplus the next day. Many people benefitted from the perks of Matt's job.

Our reliable, lanky teen was quickly and frequently recognized for being proactive. He promptly cleaned up spills, reported any issues that could impede customer satisfaction and started taking initiative in areas beyond the scope of his job description, or managerial request. Matt's name frequently adorned the staff notice board, reaping praise for going the extra mile. Matt earned *Employee of the Month* distinction more than once. The corporate employee recognition form featured Mighty Mouse flying through the air with the balloon message "You Saved the Day." A sample managerial *Mighty Memo of Praise* stated: "Thanks a million for going beyond your duties to replace all the burnt-out light bulbs in the theatre so that brightness can be restored for our guest safety."

What the note didn't mention was how Matt accomplished this task. On days off, Matt visited the theatre when in the vicinity. Daytimes were slow, with few staff on-site. Nobody paid much attention to Matt's inquisitive wanderings. On one such day Matt took replacement theatre light bulbs from the storage area and proceeded to the maintenance room. There he climbed a steel ladder, opening a hatch into the once-majestic theatre's equally cavernous attic. Then he navigated narrow catwalks with no railings, crawling on all fours and stretching over the expansive ceiling to replace burnt-out bulbs. If he'd fallen through the ceiling, it would have been about a two-story drop to the theatre seats. Knowing his actions would not have been sanctioned, Matt proudly reported his actions only upon completion of his mission.

I didn't comprehend the extent of the risk until Matt insisted on showing me his process, assuring me that nobody would mind. Reluctantly, I followed into the dingy, secluded maintenance area, still in my work clothes and high heels. He insisted I climb the ladder and poke my head through the hatch, to fully appreciate his accomplishment. Heart in my mouth, I insisted Matt stop in his tracks and only point to which bulbs he'd replaced. I made him promise to never do it again. While guests were safer due to Matt's actions, he'd put himself in harm's way.

Ever persistent, Matt wanted to expand his role. His favourite manager, Stephen, who was very well intentioned, eventually acquiesced. Our son was now assigned to change the marquee on a rotating basis with his peers. The double-sided marquee towered above the theatre on Edmonton's busiest downtown street. It rested atop a platform over the front entrance. Employees accessed the marquee from permanently attached ladders on each side. Although Matt loved changing the sign, it scared the life out of our family. Employees weren't tethered when doing the work.

"Mum, I'm perfectly safe. I just don't like it when some stupid guy driving by thinks it's funny to honk loudly and try to scare me off the ladder. Don't worry, I always hold on with my spare hand."

"Not my idea of safe and secure. I should talk to Stephen. Bet the government's Occupational Health and Safety staff would agree that Paramount needs to find a better way."

"Oh Mum, don't you *dare*—please! I'm like all the guys when I do that job and nobody's ever been hurt. It's my favourite duty and I don't want to be taken off the list."

Torn, I lived with my fears. Suppressing safety concerns, I indulged my son's joy at being treated like *one of the guys.*

Matt had the honour of changing the marquee the evening before the release of the highly touted *Pearl Harbor.* Matt was fresh in the door and taking off his coat when I answered the phone. The theatre manager, Stephen, sounded anxious to speak with Matt.

I overheard Matt say, "Oops, sorry about that." He tapped his hand on his forehead a few times and sighed. "Sure, I can do that. Yah I'll have it done before noon. Sorry—didn't mean to."

"What was that about, Matt?"

"Boy I can be such a *stupidhead*." He ignored my stern face of admonishment. "I spelled *Pearl Harbor* wrong—on both sides of the marquee. Stephen needs it fixed in the morning."

En route to work early the next morning I quickly detoured to check out the spelling error. Approaching from the east I looked up. The soaring marquee announced *Preal Harbor*. I drove another block to clearly see the west view in my rear-view mirror. Abruptly pulling over to the curb, I called Neil. He had trouble deciphering words through my gales of laughter.

Neil rushed downtown and took pictures before the spelling errors were amended. *Preal Harbor* struck me as funny, but the winner was the west-facing sign, aptly named *Peral Harbor*. Oh so true! Matt's tenure as a Paramount employee ended shortly after stepping into the world of post-secondary education, at age 19.

Matt attended two post-secondary educational programs. First, a specialized transitional vocational program, within Olds College, where he lived on campus. A couple of years later an opportunity arose to apply for an inclusive post-secondary experience in Edmonton. Matt was thrilled to be accepted at the Northern Alberta Institute of Technology, NAIT. He audited the Radio and Television Arts program. All students had the same assignments. Matt put his unique interpretation on each one.

He signed out bulky, professional camera equipment and sometimes recruited me as equipment manager when filming his favourite subjects, Edmonton city buses and the Light Rapid Transit (LRT) train system. I recall climbing unsteady terrain and wading through long grass on a hillside, listening for the train's approach.

"Here it comes! Steady the tripod, Mum. I want to shoot every bit, from the headlight coming out of the tunnel until the last car crosses the High Level Bridge. I'll edit and do my voiceover at school tomorrow." His creativity was impressive.

I fondly recall one interview assignment. The opening ceremonies for the LRT line's initial expansion were imminent. Matt knew that the inaugural run was reserved for senior project officials, politicians and the press. Calling the city, Matt made a convincing argument— as a Radio and Television Arts student he should be considered press. He wrangled a second pass for an essential resource, his equipment manager.

Matt interviewed the director of the expansion project. I turned away to hide a chuckle when the official couldn't answer a pointed question, about a recent structural challenge with the project. He respectfully directed Matt to the head engineer who provided a clear explanation. Matt shook hands with all officials and thanked each for their interview. Near the end, he caught sight of an unexpected federal Member of Parliament. Matt squeezed his way into the crowd of reporters and asked her about federal funding.

During that school year, our eager son joined a Radio and Television Arts student committee. The assignment was to explore options and consider specific proposals for a program fundraiser. Committee members would cast votes on their preferred choice.

"Wait until they hear what I've arranged. Mine will definitely be the winner."

"You've got a great option, but remember it's up to the group. Maybe they'll choose something else." Matt rolled his eyes. "Just sayin'…."

He had reached out to the organizer of the upcoming Edmonton Indy Race Car Show, a relative. The event was a hot ticket item that summer. Sheldon kindly donated a pair of tickets, providing free admittance, plus reserved front-row seats. Matt arrived at the committee meeting with a manila envelope containing an

Edmonton Indy flyer and the pair of prestigious tickets. Committee members voted and the verdict was unanimous, except for one naysayer. The prize was a pair of tickets, including free admission and drink tickets, for a student Beer Night. Matt was flabbergasted and disgusted.

"Don't they know what a good deal they've passed up? Really— choosing to get drunk over going to the Indy! And they're supposed to be smart? Dumb, dumb, dumb!"

Matt ended up awarding the Indy tickets to the third caller on a campus radio program that he hosted one Saturday evening. "At least she appreciated what she won. Stupid committee…."

I wasn't exempt from harsh judgement too. I recall a day in young adulthood when Matt was living with his roommate Fletcher. Our son called me at work requesting that I pick him up at the grocery store after his solo grocery shopping expedition. He'd bought more than he could carry. Mr. Overboard was one of his many well-deserved nicknames.

"Come on, Mum. Can't you leave work early?"

"No, Matt. You got there by bus. You can get home that way too."

"Actually, I had to take the bus *and* LRT. And big, posted signs say grocery carts aren't allowed past the parking lot. Even then I'd still need to get everything underground to the LRT and on a bus. You're not being very fair, Mum. And that's undeniably true."

"We sure see things differently. What's not fair is you interrupting my work. Taking the LRT to shop at the end of the line doesn't make sense and now you're in a pickle. I'd suggest you return some bulky items and carry what you can. With the remaining money, you can shop near home."

"What??? The buys were too good to pass up so I won't return them. Unbelievable—won't even help out your own son!"

194

"That's right. I trust you to come up with a plan. Bye." I fumed and fretted, wondering how that would turn out. Ingenuity and good luck saved the day.

Pushing the overflowing grocery cart beyond store property, Matt abandoned it amidst the others near the LRT. A kind stranger agreed to watch his items as he ran back and forth bringing his multiple purchases to the elevator. From there he descended to the LRT level. At the platform, two passengers helped him load items on the train's floor. A similar process unfolded when he got off the LRT. Unfortunately, his destination station didn't have an elevator nearby, just an escalator.

"Mum, I tossed soft stuff on the escalator near the platform. Then I ran up the stairs to take it off. Was worried the teeth from the stair treads might rip the paper towel packaging—didn't though."

"And then?"

"I piled everything beside the escalator, ran back downstairs and took the escalator up with my heavy stuff. Was sweating like a dog, so I took a short break. A kind senior citizen and his daughter stopped and helped me carry light stuff to the bus stop by the entrance. Figured a way to take only one bus. Knew it was the best choice, even though it meant a long ride home, winding through lots of areas before reaching mine."

"Sounds like quite an adventure—a needless one I might add."

"Turned out fine. Knew the bus driver. He's usually grumpy, but it was my lucky day. He shook his head in disbelief and told me not to rush getting on and off. That really surprised me."

"Probably as much as your grocery haul surprised him."

"Maybe. So glad the 7-Eleven is right beside the bus stop. The clerk Gerry watched everything, while I ran home and back again, and again. Took me five trips—that's right, five. And boy am I tired."

Such memories are typically easier to laugh about from the rear-view mirror, once everything's safely dealt with.

Matters of public and personal safety have always been important for Matt. He has never hesitated to share his observations and concerns with authority figures when opportunities arise. This pattern continued when he graduated to condo living in his early 30s. Ever vigilant about safety, he routinely apprised the building manager about concerns, no matter how minor. Luis appreciated Matt's watchfulness, patiently listened to suggestions, addressed what he could and shared concerns with the condo board. Matt continued to ponder matters.

One fall day Matt took advantage of a promotional event at McDonald's. They offered patrons the chance to discuss community concerns with a local police officer. Matt talked about building security issues and sought advice. Following up, Matt arranged and attended a productive meeting between the police and the building manager at the condo complex. Inexpensive practical strategies were identified to strengthen building security and a decal posted, designating that police have the authority to address any situation if tenants are feeling intimidated or threatened.

A few weeks later Matt was in the lobby while a condo board meeting was ongoing in the adjacent boardroom. Luis saw Matt through the window and waved him in. The condo board took the opportunity to thank Matt for his initiative.

In stark contrast to how he was judged in his initial supported independent living arrangement, in his condo complex this same man is viewed as a *proactive citizen* who is appreciated for his vigilance.

Freedom, resourcefulness and responsibility are hallmarks of growing up. Matt has collected indelible memories and a few scars while embracing the fullness of citizenship. Emancipation tests people and builds character. Why should Matt's journey be any different?

Chapter 20: In Transit Veritas

The school's call jolted my morning. It was the junior high's librarian—Mrs. Elbrond, someone we knew and trusted. "Everything okay?" I queried anxiously.

"Oh yes. Just thought you'd like to know about Matt's travels today." Mrs. Elbrond could not conceal the chuckle in her voice. "He had a bit of assistance getting here on time."

"Assistance? But he caught the bus. At least he wasn't at the bus stop when I drove by. Did something go awry en route?" Mrs. Elbrond had a soft spot for Matt so conversations with her were always open and direct.

"Sounds like he dawdled at the transit centre and missed his bus connection. One of the teachers spotted him hitchhiking near the corner. He was happy to get the lift."

"Hitchhiking? Oh, you can bet I'll be reinforcing a few things tonight. Waiting for the next bus might make him late, but will save him from his mother's wrath. Please thank the teacher for me. Hopefully this was a one-time event."

Public transit isn't renowned for its allure. However, for our son, riding the buses is as inviting and comfortable as an old slipper. Taking buses to school began once he settled into junior high. Experimenting with independent travelling reminded our family to focus on capacities. Initially this stretch felt risky, as it involved transferring buses. Like developing muscular flexibility, stretching beyond our personal comfort levels reaped benefits. Our whole family unit gained varying degrees of increased freedom.

Every morning Matt was hustled out the door and down the back lane leading to the bus stop. His independence allowed for a few minutes alone with Kate when driving her to elementary school.

With both kids at school, I headed off to work. Mission accomplished.

Looking out the bus window, our son absorbed a myriad of sights and sounds, free from life's expectations and pressures. He first experienced the soothing solace of the bus during a time of loss. My younger brother had died. I flew to be with immediate family at the funeral, on the east coast of Canada, about four thousand kilometres away. Neil and the kids stayed home, keeping me in their thoughts. Our sensitive son mourned the loss of a dear uncle, embraced by the comforting rhythm of the bus.

Adhering to school routines, Neil had sent Matt off to catch the bus. After lunch the school called to say he didn't show up for any classes. That was in the days before cell phones so Neil couldn't reach him. Matt found solace by riding the buses all day long. When our son turned up hungry at suppertime, he had processed the loss and regained emotional stability. His safe return released the gridlock that had seized our bodies and minds.

Independence with getting to and from school became routine. One day in grade eight, as Matt waited for the bus home, peers passing by stopped to bully him. Their harassment caught the eye of a vigilant bus driver heading in the opposite direction. Quickly pulling to the curb, the driver put on his four-way flashers, exited the bus and ran across the street. He yelled at the kids who scattered, then checked that Matt was okay.

Brushing the pelted snow off his jacket and face, Matt said, "I'm fine. They just like to bug me even though I'm only waiting for the bus. Thanks for chasing them away. Holy smokes, didn't know they were such fast runners!"

"I have no time or patience for hooligans. What school do you go to? I'm going to report this to your principal." When he did, Mrs. Grey noted that it occurred off school property and brushed it off as "kids being kids." Matt labelled the bus driver a hero and for many years happily reported anytime he encountered this driver on bus excursions.

By the time Matt was in senior high, his sophisticated knowledge of bus routes and schedules allowed him to explore what was happening in every part of the city. As this passion grew, Matt became a walking encyclopedia on Edmonton Transit's issues, projects and long-range planning.

Like a seasoned project manager, Matt nonchalantly informed us about every facet of the new Light Rapid Transit system, the introduction of articulating buses, seasonal route changes and the latest mobility-related enhancements to accommodate passengers. He actively participated in public consultation meetings and focus groups that sought community feedback about proposed system changes. Without fail, he was the youngest participant in such events.

Safely encapsulated in buses, Matt sat near the driver for the best view. Unless engaging the bus driver, his focus was looking out and watching communities pass by. Whenever upset, bus rides helped Matt regain equilibrium, while decompressing and seeing all parts of the city.

Throughout his late teens and into his 20s Matt enjoyed long bus rides well into the evening. Talking about risks didn't dissuade him. Hastily and bravely, Matt routinely stepped off the bus to help somebody who seemed to be in distress, whether being bullied, experiencing mobility challenges or crying in despair. This was a double-edged sword, with the potential for saviour to turn victim within moments. We've always appreciated and encouraged our son's humanity, which contributes to his value as a responsible, caring citizen. With him in control, not us, we armed him with a cell phone as soon as they became readily affordable.

Intrigued by different surroundings, Matt frequently checked out the more colourful parts of town. As evenings wore on, my calls encouraged him to head home. On one occasion I heard muttering in the background and a short reply from Matt.

"Matt, who's that you were talking to?" I tried to sound casual.

"Just a guy asking if I had loose change or a cigarette. I told him, no."

"Where are you? Doesn't sound like a good location." The concern in my voice had surfaced.

"Jeez Mum—stop worrying! I always sit near the driver so I'm safe."

"Tell me—does the driver get off the bus with you?" I snapped.

"Of course not! You know that. I get my cell phone out if there's any sign of trouble." Oh, how different our perspectives were.

"Matt, is there a corner store or gas station close by where you can wait for me to pick you up? It is getting late." I held my breath.

"Yah, there's one almost beside me. Okay I'll wait if you come right now. Hold on, hold on—no, changed my mind! See a bus coming the other way. Gotta run or I'll miss it—should be home soon. Bye."

Matt believed that jumping buses like checkers could get him home quicker. Sometimes that proved true. At other times he nabbed the last run of the night, hopping off the bus en route to the bus barns. In that stable, buses were cleaned and refuelled for the next day. A place of work for transit personnel, not visitors—usually.

Wallets and Matt have a history of parting ways—occasionally reuniting, but often not. One weekend after repeated calls to the City of Edmonton's Lost and Found department, he was assured that if cleaning staff had found the wallet, the earliest it would be turned in was Monday. It was likely a rookie staff who raised the idea of going directly to the bus barns, if the need was urgent. That was all the invitation he needed.

201

"Mum, the customer service rep said I can go ask them. Come with me, please. Probably won't let me in by myself, but maybe if I'm with you. And you know I need that wallet." What I needed was for him to stop obsessing about it.

"Okay, okay, but we'd need to go right away." I put my coffee cup down and turned around. His coat was already on. Matt was giddy at the prospect of peeking into this vast secretive warehouse space.

With a hefty tug Matt managed to open the heavy steel door. It announced our arrival with a baritone groan. The dimly lit cavernous space smelled of old wood, perfumed by diesel fumes. A transit official leaned back in his chair behind a counter to our right. Spying us, the man shot upright, tucked his book away and broadened his shoulders. Matt approached, exchanged names with Frank and stated why we were there.

"Sorry, no wallets found here. We don't get the public coming here directly. Everything we find gets sent downtown."

"I know, I go there…lots. But it's my only wallet. I lost one last month too, so my mum's not very happy." Right, blame it on me. I looked at Frank and shrugged my shoulders.

With his toes barely touching the ground, Matt leaned far over the counter. I pulled his coat collar to keep him from tumbling into Frank's domain. For my benefit, Matt cleared his throat then pointed to long rows of buses in the distance.

Frank, a keen observer, unzipped his vest of professionalism. "From that look in your eye young man, I take it you're a bus lover."

"Yes sir, that I am. Knew most buses get Sunday off, but wow—I didn't think this many. Look Mum, there's one of the new articulating buses."

Frank's demeanour softened. "I shouldn't be doing this, but it's pretty quiet at the moment." Looking around he added, "Would you like a quick tour?" Matt's eyes illuminated his face, leaving no doubt.

Matt's knowledge of the many bus models and latest features impressed our tour guide. Frank pointed out a new fare system on the latest model. "Interesting," I said.

"Not really surprising, Mum. That's probably 'cause of that bus driver who was caught stealing money from the fare box a while ago. He was charged." Looking at our guide, Matt added, "City Transit made a wise decision."

Frank's eyes bulged. In his momentary pause for words, the sound and smell of a bus engine starting up caught our attention. "Looks like it's shift change so we'd best wrap up the tour."

Frank hustled us back to the outer area. Waiting for Matt to finish his extended goodbye, I scanned the job notice board. Bus drivers, clerical positions and then...

"Matt before we go, have a look at this." I pointed out a job description for a part-time position, as a bus cleaner. I nabbed pen and paper to write down the pertinent information. Then I noticed it.

"Sorry to bother you Frank, but the qualifications don't seem to match the job description. Would you mind having a look?"

Matt pushed his glasses up his nose, studied the posting and rubbed his hands in glee. He still hadn't seen the strange part. But Frank saw it.

"Well I'll be damned. Can't explain why they'd require someone to have a driver's licence to clean a bus."

Hesitantly, I asked, "Would someone in that position ever have to move a bus, for any reason?"

"Never—and I've worked here a long time. Probably a bureaucratic screw-up. Not unusual."

"Rest assured, I can inquire. This a job worth looking into Matt?"

"Definitely! I'd love to work here. Promise you'll check into it right away?"

"First thing tomorrow morning." I used the rest of the day to strategize.

I wrote the mayor about the puzzling job posting and requested a meeting to discuss employment barriers. I was not seeking a job guarantee, but rather the opportunity to clarify, negotiate and apply if Matt met relevant job criteria. By now I knew to bring a skilled advocate along with me. Naturally the system brought an ally too—the city's head of human relations.

The mayor's directness, understanding and passion were impressive. He supported the removal of the inane driver's licence requirement and requested bureaucratic direction on how to proceed.

Squirming in his seat, the human relations director balked. The mayor's passion met its bureaucratic counterpart. The director implored the mayor not to be hasty, citing union considerations and system processes. Myopic bureaucratic mentality and persistence triumphed over justice and common sense.

The compromise was creating a bureaucratic committee to weigh all considerations—a narrow, well-trodden path, with restricted vision. Matt was offered unnecessary help to spruce up his resume. The coveted bus cleaner job description was eventually revamped and people with developmental disabilities did get to work there. Sadly, it was done in an outmoded, patronizing manner. The position was routinely filled by group-home residents. Typical employment avenues were hijacked and the job became a work program by another name. We'd have no part of that.

During Matt's protracted fixation on evening rides, I learned to trust one bus driver in particular: Norm. He was Matt's all-time favourite. Like a bloodhound, Matt sniffed out Norm's work schedule, bus

204

running-board number and route. It never took him long to track Norm down.

One wintery Saturday evening I accepted Matt's invitation to join him for an excursion on Norm's route.

"Just so you know Mum, I always sit in the front row across from Norm. You can sit there too, but by the window."

"Okay. You'll be sitting beside me?"

"Of course. I wouldn't leave you. Sitting in the aisle seat is best for talking with the driver. If someone is already in my spot, I move up as soon as they get off."

From his aisle seat, Matt leaned forward so he and Norm could readily converse. Like an observant mouse, I focused on remaining quiet, relatively undetected.

There was an easy camaraderie between the two. Conversation ebbed and flowed, covering a wide river of transportation topics. System innovations, rider and pedestrian safety, pending changes in bus routes, the retirement of old buses and construction delays with the new rail system were all discussed.

"Norm, will you learn to drive the new trains when the rail system is finally done?" Matt asked.

"Nah, I'm sticking with driving buses. Train's a whole different beast. Driver's totally separated from his passengers. I like to know who's travelling with me."

"Must say, you're fabulous at watching over all your passengers to make sure there's no trouble. I'm stoked about riding on the train and through tunnels—hope you understand. But you can count on me to still hop on your bus."

As the bus route wound deeper into the inner city, I watched the clientele change. The toll of heavy life stressors was evident on faces as people got on and off the bus. Norm took no guff and refused a few who were intoxicated. Although his exterior was gruff, he had a compassionate heart for marginalized people and their struggles. It was not unusual for people to be allowed on without bus fare. Norm wielded the bus around tight corners, honked at inattentive pedestrians, grumbled about burned-out streetlights and bantered with Matt.

Frequent stops invited both passengers and winter's chill onto the bus. My shivers were superficial and displaced by the warmth emanating from this caring, curt and cautious driver. It was a privilege to witness an exemplary sentinel of the transit system in action.

Many kind drivers have come to know Matt with his unique traits. They've let him on the bus when he's lost his bus pass, patiently waited while he's struggled to load a month's supply of grocery items or manoeuvre unexpected, awkward items on board.

During daily phone calls Matt shares excursion highlights—from encountering old childhood friends to drivers chastising passengers hogging two seats on a cramped bus. Our son's keen observation skills and his helpful nature are always on board.

One day Matt identified that a passenger had overdosed. After confirming his suspicions with another patron, he sprung into action. Taking charge, Matt asked the driver to call dispatch and pull over at a nearby drugstore. Matt ran to the pharmacy, got an overdose antidote kit and injected the man. Our good Samaritan waited until the paramedics arrived.

"Oh my God, Matt. You did that? Shouldn't you have waited?"

"Definitely not. I felt compelled—he needed Naloxone and fast! I was comfortable injecting him since I do my own insulin shots." For Matt, it was just another bus ride.

Chapter 21: Confessions

Friday evening was calm until the phone call. Our young adult had made a decision and wanted to tell me before he acted. Thinking before acting is always to be applauded with our eldest, but I was less than receptive after a draining workweek.

"Matt, your dad and I are nestled on the couch eating popcorn and watching a movie. Can't this wait?"

"Won't take long. Just thought you'd like to know I'm going to catch the bus downtown and turn myself in."

"What…what do you mean by that? Where are you and what's going on?"

"Still out with friends. Nathan's zonked from smoking too much pot. Truthfully Mum, I've been smoking some too. I'm an adult and know it's illegal so I've decided to be responsible. Going to the police. If they arrest me, I'll need to deal with it."

"Hold on a minute, Matt. That's not the best choice." Neil saw the look of terror on my face, which contradicted the controlled words escaping my tightly compressed throat. "Let me come get you right now. Then we can talk this through, at home." Tenseness consumed my being and permeated the air. Neil knew our quiet evening was over.

"Mum, you can't change my mind. I'm still going. If you want, it's okay to come with me. Pick me up at the gas station near Nathan's house. Have to promise you'll drive me to the police station, though."

"Alright, I promise. Want me to go with you or your dad? Your choice."

"Definitely you! Dad might get mad at me—or the police. Especially if they decide to put me in jail. They'd just be doing their job though."

I gave Neil a garbled synopsis, grabbed my coat and promised to keep him posted. My brain was in overdrive. How the hell could I influence the situation and keep our son safe? My stomach churned—a familiar physical symptom when risks abound and guarantees are scarce. I'd have to employ my best advocacy skills, while reining in Matt's laser-like focus to turn himself in.

Within 15 minutes, he was safely in our car. I needed to proceed with caution, to avoid treading on our son's autonomy as an adult. "Matt, I understand you feel strongly. You created this situation, but let's try to find the best way through this, together. Can I stay with you when dealing with the police?"

"Guess so, as long as they'll let you. Can't stop me from confessing though."

"I know Matt, but let's not rush to that part. I'd like to start the discussion. You jump in anytime if I say something wrong—or if you want to add something."

"Maybe…guess that's okay. Need to tell them how worried I am about Nathan. 'Cause it's true." I didn't give a damn about Nathan at the moment.

Turning off the engine in the police parking lot, I took a deep breath. "Okay, before we go, remember, I'll start first." Matt had already opened the car door, and had a foot on the ground— eager to confess. Too much so for my liking.

My warrior spirit rallied, while hoping to avoid a skirmish. Negotiation was key. After all, I'd be dealing with the police. My angel persona would take the lead.

In the doorway we passed a man exiting, while grumbling at nobody in particular. His exit fortunately left the cavernous foyer

208

temporarily empty. The officer who approached the counter was brusque. Our arrival required rising from his desk before fully settling into his chair.

Struggling to mask my worried eyes with a bright smile I said, "We'd like to discuss a matter with a police officer please." Matt was pressed up against me, doing his utmost to remain silent. His anxious breathing swirled in my ear.

"Do you have a crime to report? If so, fill out the appropriate form on the rack." Pointing to a small alcove, filled with labelled forms and a desk, he brusquely added, "You'll find what you need there—all categorized too."

Matt immediately walked over and started checking out the forms. That precious window of time provided an opportunity to massage the conversation. It was imperative to maintain a cheery demeanour. "I suspect a report isn't necessary, but talking with the duty officer would clarify that. We don't mind waiting."

Before he could respond, his phone rang and a couple walked in the door. Sighing and reaching for his phone, the officer pointed at wooden chairs lining the wall. "Alright I'll let someone know. Probably take a while." Getting past the gatekeeper was the initial step.

The new arrivals weren't so lucky and were directed to complete paperwork first. Oblivious to the new arrivals, Matt stood blocking the small alcove, with his hands on his hips. Enraptured by the rack's multiple slots, overflowing with paper, he kept scanning the array of options.

"Hey Matt" I called, patting the hard chair beside me. He turned, let the couple slip past him, then joined me in the row of seats.

Shaking his head, Matt muttered, "So many different forms, all with lots of parts." He sighed. "Still remember how my hand ached from filling out that long form when my bike was stolen. Loved that bike. Just left it for a minute...."

"I know. Disappointing we didn't ever get it back. We're waiting to talk with an officer who can decide if a form needs to be filled out. Let's hope not."

Matt got impatient when a half hour turned into 45 minutes. "I'm getting hungry." I shot him a *too bad* look. His case of the munchies wasn't on the top of my priority list. I'd planned to be sharing a quiet, relaxing evening with Neil, not strategizing at a police station.

Shuffling feet, patting his pockets and fidgeting with old magazines signalled that Matt's patience was wearing thin. "Jeez, I keep looking at the clock and time sure is moving slow. You sure it's right? Probably needs new batteries."

"Patience Matt, patience." Inwardly I pleaded for the duty officer. We were on borrowed time.

"Maybe I should just go over and find the right form to get started."

As he started to stand, the dark steel door opened. An officer stepped out and invited us into the inner sanctum. I glanced reassuringly at Matt and followed him in. Now to reassure myself.

The officer ushered us to an interview room with metal chairs and a round table. "Sorry you had a long wait. How can I help you?" He spoke with a ring of sincerity. In his early 30s, I got a good sense from this man.

"Well officer, my parents taught me that following the law is important. I'd like my mum to stay with me if that's okay."

"Not a problem," the officer said.

Matt's body relaxed and he opened his mouth. "I want to con..."

"Excuse me, officer," I interrupted, while touching Matt's arm. "My son wants to share what he's been up to with friends and discuss how to handle concerns. Right, Matt?" Confessions weren't welcome on my watch. "Tell the officer the facts and *then* there can be a discussion."

210

"Right—forgot you were going to start." Matt haltingly began. "Well officer, sometimes, like tonight, we smoke some marijuana, or pot or weed—what word do you want me to call it?"

"People call it lots of names—any of those will do." The officer leaned forward, placing his left hand under his chin. A pen and notepad were close by.

"Well even though I'm nervous I'm gonna do the right thing. Just need a second." Matt repeatedly patted and fumbled around in his pockets, leaving the officer and me bewildered. Then a smile.

"Found it—stuck in the corner!" With that, Matt pulled out a small bag, with a twist tie and plunked it on the table. "Here you go officer. You decide what to do with me."

No smile connected my eyes and mouth, just astonishment. My son, with dope in his possession? The officer turned his head slightly, and covered his mouth, suppressing the hint of a smile. He turned off the brightness in his eyes, before returning his gaze to Matt. I began breathing again.

Clearing his throat, the officer sat taller. "I'm starting by taking this bag off the table," he said authoritatively. He promptly put it on a shelf behind the table.

"Young man, you came to the police because you had an illegal substance—which you turned in. Getting it out of your possession sounds like the right thing to me. Now if you kept having dope on you that would be a different story. Is that something you plan to do?"

"No officer. I'm gonna stop, now."

"Well then, I'll let you off with a warning and some advice. Try to avoid doing things with friends that can land you in trouble. Got it?"

"Yes sir. I have a question too. How can I help my friend, Nathan? I'm worried 'cause he smokes dope a lot and doesn't want to stop. Can you make someone go to counselling or something?"

"Sorry, Matt. You're a good friend to worry, but the choice is his. I know that's not the answer you were looking for but it's the truth. I'm quite sure others are waiting to see me, so we'd best wrap it up."

He escorted us back to the foyer where at least eight people were seated, all with completed forms in hand. The officer and Matt exchanged a firm gentleman's handshake and I mouthed a huge "thank you." The heavy steel door engulfed the empathetic officer and the first couple—likely not there to confess.

Once outside Matt breathed a sigh of relief. "Mum, I was scared but knew it was the right thing to do."

"And I knew it was right for me to tag along. Let's head home; I'm hungry now too. Don't worry, you'll get to start the next talk."

"Huh? What talk?"

"With your dad…." I added casually, stifling the urge to giggle.

An unexpected detour delayed that conversation. Celebrating the birth of Matt's first honourary niece took precedence. Eventually sitting at the kitchen table, our son had his opportunity to confess all.

With big doe eyes he posed the question. "So am I in trouble?" Neil's hazel eyes softened.

"You know Matt, growing up involves making your own decisions, trying new things and taking responsibility. You did all three. This time it worked out okay, but some decisions can go terribly wrong—and fast! If you're ever in doubt, ask yourself: is this something a good man might do? That's worked well for me." He gave us that familiar grin. "Well, at least most times. Hungry?"

212

Chapter 22: Justice on the Job

Intolerance and justice coexisted under one roof; introductions just hadn't been made yet. Working limited shifts at a local movie theatre for two years had whetted Matt's appetite for more. He was sniffing out other employment opportunities.

Matt stopped at our local drugstore's customer service desk. As usual he checked the employee's nametag. He badly wanted a personalized nametag.

"'Scuse me, Kate. Funny, that's the same name as my sister, but I usually call her Katie. Since he's probably already had lunch can you please page the manager on duty? Only need him for a minute."

My designated role was to keep walking. Matt's slouched shoulders conveyed the answer as I half-heartedly scanned the store flyer.

"Don't give up, Matt. Keep looking close to home. That way you can get to and from work easily."

"Why didn't I think of that before, Mum? Let's head to Safeway!"

We'd shopped at this grocery store since Matt was a baby. Many store staff knew Matt, if not by name, then by sight. I browsed the apple selection, which kept me within sight of Matt at the customer service counter. I picked tart apples for Neil to make a pie.

"Vic, customer waiting at the service desk," resounded through the store. Within a few minutes a man appeared, wearing a white shirt and black tie. I moved to the bananas for a better vantage point. The confident and professional-looking man respectfully shook Matt's hand before returning to his office. Matt tried strolling over to the produce section, but the spring in his step denoted something promising.

"Guess what—I have a job interview tomorrow! It's with Vic, the store manager. He's really nice. Think I'll wear black dress pants. That's what Vic had on."

So began almost four years of work as a courtesy clerk. Matt always prided himself on good customer service. Having a penchant for helping, it was a challenge for Matt to focus solely on core courtesy clerk tasks. Vic routinely and patiently reinforced staying on task.

"Matt, you're a good grocery packer. Your bags aren't too heavy and you protect fragile items like eggs." Vic paused to make sure Matt was listening. "I know customers sometimes ask for your help, but when possible please direct them to the customer service desk. So, tell me the three main parts of your job."

"Pack groceries, pick up red shopping baskets left at the tills and return buggies from the parking lot. But I'm always able and willing to take on other responsibilities, especially when the store's quiet."

Matt was elated whenever customer service staff assigned tasks beyond his three mundane duties. He loved returning items to their shelves during slow periods. I'd occasionally see our son scooting down the aisle on the back of a shopping cart, while returning items and enjoying a few minutes of freedom. At the checkout, Matt engaged customers, commenting on their healthy choices and tasty treats. He injected lightness into customers' days and many knew him by name. Highly perceptive to individual struggles, Matt routinely offered carry-out services to seniors, people with mobility challenges and young mums herding small children.

Generally, he was recognized as a very hard worker with a strong customer service focus. Yet there were challenges. Like many people with developmental disabilities, Matt lacks awareness of personal space and social nuances. This became evident during quiet periods when he dutifully checked tills to ensure each cashier was well stocked with supplies. His sudden presence and quick moves in tight quarters initially startled some cashiers. Without warning, he spontaneously reached across the open till to replace a permanent marker. At other times he unexpectedly and silently crouched down

214

by the cashier to replenish grocery bags. After one or two such encounters, most cashiers relaxed and appreciated his attentiveness.

It only takes one person to put things off balance. Just as Matt presented in a unique way, there was one cashier who stood out. She exuded negativity, wore a perpetual frown and was curt with customers. Her disposition was the antithesis of her sweet-sounding name, Violet. I'd consciously avoided her till for years, preferring a longer line-up than exposure to the perpetual dark cloud that enveloped her workspace.

It was ironic that as the union's shop steward, Violet was the only staff who openly rebuffed Matt. She made no effort to accommodate Matt's differences or understand his unique contribution to the workplace. Her disdain was abundantly clear— Matt did not belong. Confident in her rights under the union, she insisted that Matt not invade her space to replace grocery bags, pick up garbage or have anything to do with her. She erected a high-voltage electric fence of intolerance around her work space whenever Matt was on shift.

This confused and stressed our son. "Why does Violet hate me? Sure don't think I've done anything wrong. She won't let me get *any* supplies for her till—none, zero, zilch. I've even seen customers have to wait while she went to get more bags. I could have done that."

I struggled to conceal my rage at the injustice. "Sorry, Matt, I can't explain it. But it's important for you to stay clear. She's like a grenade that's easy to blow up."

Neil and I met with the supportive store manager. Vic respectfully listened to our concerns, while almost imperceptible twitches danced across his raised shoulders. Like tempting a dog to the end of its tether, Violet knew exactly how far she could stretch and distort her rights under the union. Vic lacked concrete grounds to take action, so her intolerance trumped respect. No one was going to trample on her rights, but she was fine with emotionally stomping all over our son's. I could only imagine that her life was probably quite troubled. That's as charitable as I could ever get.

Violet's work presence made Matt intimidated and nervous. When shifts overlapped, we counted down the hours, hoping distance would keep the tension at bay. One quiet evening shift, Violet pulled the pin. Matt was gazing into space as he often does when daydreaming or perplexed. Looking toward the front entrance hoping for customers, his scope included Violet's workstation. Her till was nearest the store entrance. Violet abruptly declared that our son was staring at her and lodged a harassment charge with the union.

The next day, Vic called Matt into his office. "Matt, whenever an employee lays a charge with the union, there are steps that we always have to go through."

"But I didn't..."

"Matt, I need to stop you there. We'll set up meetings to get a better understanding of what happened. Until then we can't talk about it. I know this is stressful and I'll have meeting times arranged by tomorrow. It's fine to bring your parents when we meet with you. Try not to worry."

Not only was Violet the union shop steward, but also a long-term, permanent employee. Matt was a casual part-time employee in an entry position, who presented as being "different." The layers of disadvantage weighed heavily on our hearts and minds.

Neil and I were outraged at being pulled into an insane David and Goliath battle. It took all our strength to present a calm front to our bewildered son. All we wanted was tolerance and justice.

On the morning of the dreaded formal interview, Matt made an announcement at breakfast. "I want you both at the meeting, but hope you drop me off a half hour early. I want to visit with John and Sheryl first."

Matt was particularly fond of both department managers who obviously cared about him too. And so he fortified himself for the meeting, nurtured by supportive colleagues, not just Mum and Dad. At the appointed hour, Matt met us at the store entrance. He bravely walked the stairs to Vic's office with a parent on each side.

The meeting was brief and respectful. Both management and the union rep asked Matt straightforward questions. He gave simple answers, providing explanations upon request. Neil and I assisted with reframing questions when we sensed a need for clarification by any party. Both the union representative and management quickly concluded that Matt did nothing wrong. The grievance was dismissed and the issue officially considered closed. We breathed a collective sigh of relief and celebrated with ice cream.

Violet found it hard to swallow the grievance results. She remained disgruntled and perhaps provoked. The pre-existing work tension was ripe for festering.

One day when shopping, Sheryl nabbed me as she stocked shelves. "I'm so glad that union ruling cleared Matt," she said. "You know, a bunch of us were prepared to file our own union grievance if things went sideways. Glad we didn't have to—sure would have, though." With a wink and a smile she carried on with her duties.

Late one afternoon after a shift, Violet met Lisa, a recently hired cashier in the staff room. "Welcome aboard…I guess. Fair warning though, you'll be stuck with that damn weirdo kid as your courtesy clerk. I'm so sick of him," Violet muttered.

"Oh, I've worked a few shifts now. Who do you mean? Not Matt?"

"Yah, kid gives me the creeps. Always messing around the tills."

"Well customers sure love him. He's been welcoming to me too; keeps my shopping bags stocked up so I don't have to get them."

Violet sputtered something unintelligible. Lisa wasn't the sympathetic audience she was hoping for.

"If it was up to me they wouldn't hire people like *that*." As Lisa silently scrambled to leave the room, Violet threw a closing barb, "He's such a re…"

She abruptly amputated the word, sensing a looming presence. Looking up, Violet saw Sheryl standing in the staff room door.

With her hands on her hips and a screwed-up face, Sheryl said "Wanna finish what you were starting to say?"

Violet shrugged her shoulders and reached for her coat. She knew better than to cross swords with Sheryl.

With eyes afire, Sheryl added, "Changed your mind? Then let me say it for ya. Matt's a *reeeally* hard worker, who's kind, customer focused and a valued employee. Certainly can't say that for some others. Air's pretty foul in here—makes me want to puke!" Shooting a final glare, Sheryl turned and left the room.

Lisa abruptly followed. "Omigod Sheryl, thanks for saving me from her vile tirade—made my skin crawl. Can't imagine how she makes Matt feel."

"You're right. I'm not sure what can be done, but it needs to stop. One of these days her foul-mouthed yappin' will be her downfall."

Sheryl was not prepared to let this slide. She sought out the manager. "Vic, you got a minute?"

Now on high alert, Vic encouraged feedback, fine-tuned his own ears to sonar mode and listened. A slip-up was inevitable. Then the weekend arrived….

I dropped Matt off for a shift. He was immediately greeted by a senior staff inside the front entrance.

"Good man, right on time. Need you to come out back with me."

"Okay. Probably should sign in first."

"Can do that later. Quickly now Matt, let's go. I think John's working today." She quickly ushered him to the store's rear warehouse, where deliveries are made.

"Sounds like something's wrong. Am I in trouble?"

"Matt, you're fine. Just stay put and Vic will come by to explain shortly."

Our son loved rare opportunities to experience this bustling area, where delivery trucks arrived, products were unloaded and boxes crushed. But today he was totally in the dark and worried. Crossing his arms, he paced, his body knotted with stress. Suddenly the swinging doors opened wide. Vic appeared and immediately read the dread on Matt's face.

Gently he said "Matt let's go into John's back office for a minute—I have news." Once behind the closed door, Vic leaned against the desk and said, "Your problems with Violet are over. She's no longer working at this store, effective immediately."

"Oh…is that my fault, Vic? I'm sorry if I…"

"No, not your fault at all, Matt."

We were never given details, nor did we ask. However, it was clear that Vic's attentiveness paid off. Perhaps an unsuspecting Violet spouted off within Vic's earshot. Whatever the spark, it was documented. Ensuing action was quick and decisive. Violet's behaviour was likely considered discriminatory under the Labour Code, giving Vic grounds to take decisive action.

Violet was swiftly escorted from the premises and transferred to another store. This drama was unfolding in Vic's office as Matt's shift was about to begin. Our son had been caringly whisked away to avoid entanglement.

"Like I never have to worry about her again? Vic, that feels like a miracle."

"She's gone. Now off you go young man, your shift is starting." With a smile he added, "Have a good day and remember..."

"Don't you worry, Vic. I've got it covered—bagging, red baskets and buggies." Justice had prevailed.

Section 3· Balance, Strength and Accountability

Gaining Perspective

Chapter 23: The Gift

Words of awe flowed from my heart. "Well, hello there." Her silent presence enveloped me, evoking a "love at first sight" response.

The sculpture was new, soaring regally from a shelf in the chiropractor's office. Forged steel wings seemed to flutter upward into the air, as if turning solid metal into wind. I ached for such steely resolve to manage ongoing challenges and conflicts, in my quest for ordinary.

Fixated on this compact beauty, I eagerly awaited my chiropractor's arrival. Dr. Tash's smiling face appeared and I immediately launched into questions, trying not to sound all-consumed—yet I was.

"Kevin, I can't take my eyes off your masterpiece," I said, while lying prone and pointing towards the shelf. "Where did you get such a remarkable creation?"

Tossing his head towards his colleague's adjoining office he said, "Actually, it was a gift from Dan. He's an amazing artist."

"Seriously, Dan? It's spellbinding. Think he might consider commissioning another?"

"Dan's creativity is boundless and his range of work is far reaching."

His colleague's other creations weren't on my mind. "Does the sculpture have a name?"

"Don't recall the mention of a name." Kevin's soft voice brought the conversation to a close. "Roll over now and I'll work on your front."

His skilled hands gently and adeptly aligned my body. As a chiropractor he was gifted at fusing his hands, heart and ears. He had absorbed it all—my words and palpable connectedness to this artwork.

After the treatment Kevin asked me to wait a moment. Lost in thought, I automatically put on shoes, picked up my purse and stood up. Standing silently, a few feet in front of me, his lips curved into a Mona Lisa smile. I was puzzled.

Reaching behind his back, Kevin revealed the coveted sculpture tenderly saying, "I think this more appropriately belongs to you."

Awe flooded every chamber of my heart. Inadequate words surfaced.

"What? Oh, I couldn't. Dan handcrafted this sculpture specifically for you! Admittedly I love it, but…"

He interrupted, gently touching my arm. "I want you to have it. Your strength and courage are reflected in her…it's a perfect match." He didn't budge.

I spontaneously threw my arms around him in gratitude, kissed his cheek and tried to hold back tears. "Well then, she needs a fitting name to reflect her soaring spirit. I'll call her *Warrior Angel*."

Kevin's smile broadened as he opened the door for his next appointment—my teenage son, Matt. I stepped out of the office, averting my eyes. I had to hide brewing tears. I felt the burn of admonishment as he brushed past, eager to shake the hand of his cherished chiropractor. "Morning, Dr. Tash. Sorry my mum's put you a bit behind schedule. Don't worry, I've waited patiently." Typically, Matt was highly perceptive to emotional states. Momentarily, he was oblivious to my fragility. I needed to get a grip and fast.

Swiftly crossing the waiting room, I melted into a corner chair, placing the sculpture at my feet. I tried flipping mindlessly through magazines as a distraction. But my eyes, like the eyes of a lover, kept being drawn to the sculpture. This intense attraction was hard to process—at least initially.

The angel's outspread wings vibrated with power, brandishing a broadsword. Heat patterns in the metal illuminated the energy bursting from her core, like chakras given form. The gradations of steel captured a spirit that ranged from glittering light to brooding darkness.

For me, her rootedness to the earth suggested strength, courage, determination and resilience. The raised sword symbolized her preparedness to spare no effort in life's battle for justice, understanding and inclusion. Each finely imposed feature exuded the message of unsentimental love, a love tested by unyielding endurance.

My dense clouds of perplexity dissipated and I brightened, now comprehending the attraction. *Warrior Angel*'s duality speaks to lifelong advocacy for our son. In seeking an ordinary life for our son, duality is hardwired into my soul. Vigilance and timing are critical. My persona can change at Batman speed. Formidable wings are at the ready, to either swoop into action or savour rare, sensuous moments of relaxation.

Unlike this angel of forged steel, my core can swiftly dissolve into moulded jelly. At such times the power of my convictions keeps me plodding forward, trembling with each step. At other times, my tenacity firmly resides in limbo, on sabbatical until I regain the stamina to take one more stride.

Matt's presence abruptly shook my tangled web of thoughts. "Mum, are you okay?" He looked renewed by his treatment but concerned that he'd startled me. In half a heartbeat his focus shifted, captured by the mound of steel at my feet.

"What the heck is that? Definitely wasn't there before. Did someone forget it? I could ask Deb." Hearing her name, the receptionist looked up. I smiled and shook my head. I had this under control. "Sure looks heavy, Mum. Can I pick it up?"

224

Touching Matt's arm gently paused the blitz of curiosity. "All good questions. Actually, it's mine—amazingly a gift from Dr. Tash. Who would have thought? Let's talk about it over an early lunch. Interested?"

"Sure! Saw a flyer yesterday about a new restaurant somewhere near here. Even mentioned grand opening specials. Bet I can find it quick, so let's go. Ready, Mum?"

Standing up, I reached for the prized treasure, snatching it just ahead of Matt's nimble outstretched fingers. We both smiled and I gave a playful nudge. "Hey buddy, that belongs to me."

I absorbed *Warrior Angel*'s weight and pervasive energy. My palm and fingers perfectly encircled her waist—as if customized for me. In turn, her spirit grasped me just as firmly, in oh so many ways.

Chapter 24: Stand by Me

Brittle, like dried-out kindling, our family could be readily snapped and set ablaze. Warm-hearted friends and family—clearly allies—witnessed our relentless pressures, from the outside looking in. We needed strength from those who knew it up close and personal—other families who lived with the complexities of disability and vulnerability.

Broken families swirl like cinders in the wind, remnants of their former robust selves. To avoid this fate, we needed to grasp a strong branch. It came through my work connections with the organization formerly called Alberta Association for Community Living (AACL), currently Inclusion Alberta.

A strong advocacy organization, AACL supports families and individuals with developmental disabilities who crave ordinary lives of inclusion, in community. One day at work, their CEO approached me during a meeting break. AACL had started an innovative pilot project to train families in advocacy. The Family Leadership Series was designed to be intensive, free of all costs and provide quality childcare as needed. The bonus feature was international gurus, as guest speakers. Bruce wanted Neil and me to consider it. He didn't downplay the commitment. That was never his style.

"Really—sessions run all weekend long?" He let my rhetorical question hang. "Five weekends spread over a few short months is a big ask, but I'm intrigued. I'll talk with Neil and let you know later this week."

A parent himself, Bruce epitomized a fierce warrior angel for inclusion. He unwaveringly challenged systems while standing solidly with families who needed to be braced. Representing AACL in government meetings with stakeholders, Bruce routinely excused himself during discussion of important provincial matters, to address urgent matters. Some of my colleagues bristled when he left, yet inwardly I smiled. Whenever I caught a snippet of the issue, it typically involved a family in crisis. Family needs always superseded system needs. I loved knowing such a powerful and articulate champion was in our corner, as *one of us*. With Bruce as co-facilitator of the upcoming advocacy training, Neil and I decided to hop on board.

The advocacy training overflowed with nourishment, enriching every family. Foregoing precious weekends was far outweighed by learning opportunities and the development of a deeply rooted advocacy network.

The awkwardness of strangers dissipated almost immediately. Parents shared the common experience of being dismissed, typically by professionals thinking they somehow were privy to insights that eluded us. Yet it is the parents who live the experience, each and every day, whether we feel up to it or not. What fellow advocates celebrated as success is readily judged by others as mundane. Emotional stories gushed freely, into the ocean of acceptance.

"I've worked hard to build on my daughter's capacity to have a so-called *normal* life, involved in typical community life," the mother of a young girl said. "Then the system has the nerve to suggest that being so engaged might indicate she really doesn't have a disability. I could scream!" The older woman in the next chair reached over and gently rubbed her back. Words weren't needed.

"You get punished on every front," one father added. "We simply want our children to be welcomed in the world as valued, contributing citizens. Every human being has quirks—my son too. He deserves to feel the warmth of belonging. And that warmth radiates from positive actions, not empty words." Heads bobbed in agreement.

An introverted mum found the courage to speak. "Her brother routinely gets invited to a birthday party." She paused and the group gave her space. "Invitations for Joan are rare and usually tokenism. She gets so excited, but when I pick her up she's standing on the fringe—a lonely observer." Her words trailed off, her energy spent. Someone pointed out that our children being invited to a birthday party was usually a cause for celebration. This discussion evoked a strong memory for me.

"One year I invited Matt's grade three classmates to his birthday party—all nice kids. But even then, Matt seemed like an outsider in his own home. He was the centre of attention *only* when he was opening gifts. All boys were polite and physically present, but emotionally unaware of Matt's marginalization."

It made me ponder when awareness of marginalization typically enters one's consciousness. Too late for sure. Global indifference to marginalized populations reinforces that the germination process sorely needs to be accelerated, for humanity's sake.

The advocacy series was like basic training for guerrilla warfare. Guest speakers and facilitators addressed system survival skills, diversion tactics, hand-to-hand *combat* strategies and when to call upon the troops. We were drilled to expect the unexpected. Examples illustrated how the powerful system had the means and motive to abruptly change the rules of engagement, with rationalizations at the ready. Recruits in this underground network of revolutionaries bonded deeply, while training primarily for solo missions, on behalf of our devalued loved ones.

Bruce shared a key strategy that resonated for all participants. "When the rest of the world says that you are mad, think of this group—the army on your shoulder that understands, and has your back." That enduring message has enabled me to be strong in many stressful situations. An example was when I defended my truth about the student awards ceremony, standing up to Matt's indignant senior high principal.

Every family within this collective band recognized the warrior angel sword at their feet. All consciously picked up the heavy, yet mighty weapon to help defend a vulnerable loved one. New recruits and renowned generals on the battlefield—all enriched by the experience that nurtured, strengthened and emboldened us to seek better.

Much like an intensive university course, each advocacy module was jam-packed. Friday evenings were warm-ups, reconnecting and taking an initial dip into heavy agendas. Saturday and Sunday were the full-tilt boogie. Our skilled facilitators deepened our understanding about the layers of political and bureaucratic processes, issues, challenges and strategies.

Seasoned advocates shared personal strategies to reduce the sting of judgement. One mother taught us to reframe "stubborn bitch" into "determined advocate." Another shared her standard response to slander. "You call me a bitch…like that's a bad thing." Everyone hooted, relishing being cocooned with kindred spirits. One wise parent wrote: "The energy for our leadership comes from the broken places in our hearts."

As a network we laughed, hugged and consoled—bonded as a *family of the heart*. Dedicated family members attended from all over Alberta. Neil and I were grateful that most sessions were in Edmonton, close to our home. We finished each weekend bone weary, but enlightened and strengthened in knowledge and conviction.

Facilitators reminded us that professionals built the Titanic and an amateur built the ark. Some matters are too important to be left to the professionals—the fate of vulnerable loved ones for sure. Families learned strategies to improve effectiveness when arm-wrestling with powerful systems. Fulfilling the dual role of parent and government insider, I concurred with the overviews presented. One strong message bore repeating: "systems always have a smile on their face and a gun in their pocket."

I was grateful that my government employer, the Persons with Developmental Disabilities (PDD) program, had earned an enviable reputation for being progressive and innovative. Safeguards were in place and consumer feedback was welcomed. Shortly before the PDD provincial policy was officially released, my office asked for final feedback, from straight-shooting parents. As program staff, we'd become too enmeshed in revisions to recognize when information was muddled or missing. An open-minded program, with no gun in sight.

One father, George, was a particularly vocal advocate. As we wrapped up our fruitful session, I teased him. "Knew we could count on you to give your honest opinion and not hold anything back." I winked and picked up my documents.

"Think so, do you? Not really."

That got my attention.

"I've got lots riding on maintaining a good relationship with you guys. What my daughter gets for services is ultimately in your control. My other kids were worried when I mentioned I'd be giving feedback. Lots of warnings to keep my emotions in check. In the end it looks pretty decent—for government policy, that is." George smiled, saluted and left.

I sat down, taken aback. How could I have been so blind to his risk? I'd become too engrossed, scanning policy through my governmental rose-coloured glasses.

George sent a follow-up email the next day. "I find walking the talk of inclusion elusive at best. You hear it all the time, but it's rare in practice. I'm counting on you to put Alberta's good policy intentions into practice. I'll be watching."

I wrote back, "George, rest assured I'll do my absolute best to oversee implementation. I value knowing advocates like you will point out when good intentions go astray. Hopefully we won't encounter many hiccups."

Soon after implementation of PDD's provincial policy, I travelled across Alberta, meeting with regional audiences, primarily families. The policy reflected what families told us in no uncertain terms.

I began by reading the policy framework's foundation principle; a product of extensive consultation with families across all regions: "Individuals, with the assistance of their families and friends, are the

230

'primary' source for identifying what is best for themselves and what kinds of support they require."

An advocate immediately challenged me, sounding frustrated. "Susan, like many here, I gave up precious time to participate in that consultation process. Yes, the principles are good. Initially I was really optimistic, but not so much now."

Somehow, I felt George's wariness in the room. Leaning on the podium, I put my chin in my hand, saying "I hope you'll tell me why."

"Gladly," she said, pausing to consider her words. "For starters, there's still close scrutiny of families and the legitimacy of our visions."

I sensed that this was a budding strong advocate, someone new to me. I needed more. "As a representative of the *policy puzzle palace*, that's an important message to hear—and understand. Please don't leave me hanging...." Inside, I was cheering her on.

A voice in the crowd said "Go for it, Linda—we're all behind you." Ah, a familiar refrain.

My eyes pleaded for her honesty.

"Okay, here goes. Families know we have to be accountable—within reason, of course." Stopping to take a breath, Linda dove in deeper. "What our families find missing is government accountability. Easy for you to say policies are flexible and families have power. Negotiating our personal visions is where we encounter roadblocks." She seemed to be standing taller now, having spoken boldly and conquered the jitters.

"Linda, it likely won't come as a surprise that such implementation concerns were consistently raised during our consultations. Based on those concerns we adopted supplemental principles, to guide regional practices. I'm hoping you can clarify where you're encountering roadblocks."

"Sure can. Our region has adopted its own rules and takes a hard stance on any proposal that looks *different*. Many families here are already lined up to plead their case to an appeal board."

Nods in the crowd reinforced that this woman was a spokesperson for many.

"Susan, do you have any idea how exhausting that is?"

Biting my tongue, I stuck to my role as provincial program representative. "I can only imagine that appeals are time-consuming and very stressful."

"Yes, and it's *needless* stress. The principles have no teeth. Policy words sound nice, but they get lost when we negotiate. Our proposals are measured against the restricted menu of services the region actually funds. Creative approaches aren't valued, just conformity. Feels like we've been duped."

Thunderous applause exploded. This reticent woman had turned into a firecracker before my eyes. If not a recent graduate of Family Leadership training, then an excellent candidate and advocacy role model.

"Clearly many of you feel a disconnect. I'm perplexed and can't speak to regional processes." Turning to my regional colleague, I said, "Aster, can you shed some light?" I sat down, eager to take in every wiggly word.

Smiling, the regional representative used bureaucratic jargon, stressing how each case was judged on its own merit and offering to talk privately with individuals after our session. While her lips moved, families' eyes glazed over and her message bounced off walls. I was the first to nab her after the session.

"Aster, what's going on? Program principles are abundantly clear, but even I'm struggling to see how your processes align. The crowd's sure not feeling any love."

"Our region supports the program principles and wants to encourage innovation. But budget management is an issue, so we adopted clearer funding parameters."

My lax mouth and knitted eyebrows conveyed shock and disapproval.

"Sorry Susan, but reality is reality. Principles and policy are vague and open to interpretation. And they don't specify what regions *can't* do. So we've adopted clear regional practices."

Finishing with a Cheshire cat grin, Aster turned away to greet a family with a hollow hug. Yes indeed, my own government system had a smile on its face and a gun in the pocket. Many fingerprints were on that gun, including mine—intentional or not.

Every skilled and seasoned warrior I've ever encountered routinely experiences such system struggles. And none of us are naïve enough to think it'll ever disappear. We all started as young, green saplings needing light and the protection of strong, majestic trees. Over decades we become mature trees in a forest—bearing the traits of strength, stature and endurance. Providing shelter for others is natural—part of giving back.

Long, flexible branches taught us about bending with the wind, to survive gale-force winds, and reduce risks of extensive damage. Every scar and twisted limb tells a story. Trunk wounds remind us of wind storms that ripped protective bark, exposing raw wood. Time and nutrients conducted the repair. Roots have continuously spread, deep and wide, intertwining with others sharing the forest floor. Advocacy networks sustain each other through times of drought, wind and rain. Some connections are far in distance, but never in heart. United we stand.

Chapter 25: Battlefield Reflections

The formidable steel masterpiece pierces my soul during dinner every night. A priceless and cherished gift, she epitomizes her name, *Warrior Angel*. Centre stage in the dining room display case, the sculpture sits at eye level directly across from me. Exuding relentless courage and energy, by contrast I am keenly aware of my every inadequacy as an advocate for our vulnerable son. While my spirit embraces the angel's fierce and loving duality, on a deeper level, the comparison feels ludicrous. Like a magnet, the sculpture lures dinner guests with her radiating presence. This night's no exception.

"That's an amazing piece! Definitely one of a kind." I reached into the cabinet and handed it to my friend, Patti.

"Omigod it's heavy—just like the proverbial weapon in a murder mystery. Where'd you get it?"

The story behind this gift always intrigues. As friends often do, Patti innocently launched into memories from Matt's childhood and young adulthood. I'd rather sidestep such discussions.

"Love how you booked a meeting with the mayor about employment barriers for people with disabilities. Pretty gutsy of you."

Smiling, I reclaimed the sculpture and pulled out Patti's chair with my free hand. She took my cue.

Facing the display case rather than our guests, I said, "Unfortunately, the mayor's good intentions didn't bear fruit." Returning the sculpture to her place of honour, the weight of all she embodies almost buckled my knees. "Okay, let's get this meal started! Interested in sampling Neil's homemade bread?"

"Of course. Wish my husband could cook like yours." Reaching for the bread, Patti returned to churning up memories, "Still remember the time you called the principal's bluff. But my all-time favourite…"

Squirming, I interrupted. "Ah, glory days of old. Colourful stitches in life's tapestry—God that sounds philosophical! Allen, how about filling my wine glass?"

Patti's perceptive husband, Allen, gazed into my eyes as he poured. "I protest. You dismiss too readily all the brave stances you've taken for Matt. As parents, you've both battled to get regular opportunities like all other kids on the block." With twinkling eyes, he raised his glass. "Deserves a toast to stellar parenting."

My heart demanded I clarify. "Being stellar is akin to a shooting star, bright and memorable, yet short-lived. Right, hon?" Neil's smile caressed me. Allen cocked his head and theatrically swept his hand open, an invitation to explain. I decided to share an analogy from a fellow advocate.

"Families are like punching bag clowns. Routinely get knocked down but always come back at you. Fast or slow, depends on how much air they hold." Low on energy, words faded. "I must admit, my air supply's been sorely depleted. Retired from most battles these days, conserving energy for crucial issues."

I felt like a sheep masquerading in wolf's clothing when people recalled "glory days." It's difficult to maintain a façade of confidence and vitality. My abundant supply of stamina had been drained. Increasingly relying on fumes, there was no refuelling station in sight.

Over decades, both personally and professionally, I cultivated the courage to question, challenge and combat systems as needed. Like gravity, battle fatigue pulled me down, crumbling resilience into dust. Until my last breath, I'll weigh in and stir the pot for inclusion of devalued populations, whether in the boardroom, community events or family gatherings. Efficacy may waver, yet my resolve's rock solid.

Our daughter, Kate, recalls me teaching her: "Labels are for jam jars, not people." A lesson she's passing on to our grandchildren.

A delicate crisscrossed pattern of hairline cracks adorns my timeworn sword. Excavating below this fractured surface reveals harsh realities. The once mighty steel sword has been pitted by the rust of time. Yet, pockmarks of regrets, frustration, impatience and sheer exhaustion don't overshadow pride that comes from accomplishments.

The much-admired sculpture is impervious to worldly penetration. I am not. Prolonged exposure to life's fiery elements has toughened and scarred the relentless determination of my youth. *Warrior Angel* radiates perfect poise on a steel pedestal of virtue. I've reached far, sometimes grasping the golden ring, other times falling far, far short. Or so it feels.

During Matthew's childhood we were a poster family for inclusion. It all seemed within our grasp until life unfolded and adulthood was on the horizon. Over time we lost our grip and falls became frequent—typically swift, painful and often public. I sought refuge by wedging into tight crevices of withdrawal. Every deep slide into internal exile stemmed from being overwhelmed and exhausted. Apathy or denial never played a role, yet I suspect some professionals perceived it that way.

I recall the time a micro-burst of energy helped me squeeze out of my dark sanctuary. I pulled out the reminder letter and booked that overdue specialist's appointment. Perfect timing; there had just been a cancellation.

"Mrs. Dunnigan, I see it's been awhile since Matthew's last appointment. Given his foot structure and associated balance issues, I can't stress enough the importance of maintaining a regime for regular follow-up. Naturally that includes routine podiatry."

"I understand," I uttered, striving to make my voice audible. Every muscle tensed, pleading for a full body massage—as if that would happen. Self-care was always last on the list.

"Mrs. Dunnigan?" The doctor held out a prescription. "This is for badly needed orthotics. Your son's current shoes are showing signs of significant wear. Good-quality shoes maximize effectiveness. I presume he's routinely seeing a physiotherapist too."

The doctor's underlying whiff of judgement reinforced my guilt for not keeping on top of all things important. Like a wide-mouthed funnel, my reclaimed energy vanished completely, before reaching the parking lot. The confines of that recently relinquished crevice beckoned me already.

"Can I see the orthotics prescription, Mum? Goin' to get those new shoes today?"

"Not yet, Matt. Need to get you back to school and me back to work." Mac and cheese would be on the menu for a while.

Skirmishes were easier before Matt's time clock struck adulthood. Until then I had authority and control by virtue of being his mum and legal guardian. On Matthew's 18th birthday, he gained legal rights as an adult. Parental control was snuffed out like the candles on his cake. Life twisted and became more complex.

In Matt's early adulthood, I recall a colleague gingerly broaching the subject that puzzled many. "I don't understand, Susan. Your policy work focuses on inclusion and your heart's clearly there too. So why choose one of the most conservative agencies to support Matt?"

Smiling at her forthrightness, I responded, "How long you got...? In a nutshell, the apartment's close to home, the agency's venturing into independent living and their newly adopted rhetoric aligns with inclusion. We got the last apartment and rent's affordable. So we're holding hands and leaping across the abyss. Hoping that practice lives up to promise and compatibility reigns." Major fail number one—they dumped us.

As is typical in many families, oversight is my role. I am the glue who repairs family ruptures. With a loved one as vulnerable and complex as our son, ruptures are ongoing. From multiple seeping droplets needing dabs of glue, to tossing buckets at full-blown geysers, we've been there. I don't claim to fly solo, but I am the first responder and always on call.

I've always been an ambassador for collaboration, social justice and inclusion. The pragmatic and deeply emotional sides of my brain strive to work separately and in sync, depending on each circumstance. A near impossible balancing act, I've been besieged on all fronts. In times of distress, solace came only by shutting my eyes at night, retreating into rest and privacy.

Being well trained and educated, I'd once been confident in my craftsmanship to ensure an ordinary life of inclusion. After all, I was a professional social worker, working in the field of disability, attended workshops with international gurus, experienced intensive advocacy training and enjoyed a strong emotional support network. And yet, it was still beyond my control. My heart goes out to the throngs of families seeking ordinary, who lack an equivalent toolbox of resources. Without allies, chances of survival on the battlefield are slim.

When confidence erodes and energy evaporates, my spirit retreats, becoming a mere shadow of my once strong warrior angel persona. Yet, regardless of energy's ebb and flow, my ocean-deep capacity to comprehend and relate to Matt remains constant.

More than anyone, I appreciate his inherent struggles to build on life experiences and reap the knowledge that comes from natural consequence. Knowing critical life lessons may never be fully absorbed and integrated can leave me lost in the wilderness, judged as the overcompensating, gullible mother. In reality, I am my own harshest critic.

As a mother, I try to remain aware, open-minded and prepared for anything. Matt's ingenuity, resilience and knowledge about passionate pursuits routinely amaze me. Equally amazing is how basic daily living considerations readily escape him, well into adulthood. Surprise and exasperation are my ever-present conjoined twins.

Understanding our son's complexities and human frailties doesn't exempt me from judging. It's easy to add my barbs to the frustrated choir, demanding that as an adult he *do better*. I've readily succumbed to the urge to skewer.

"For God's sake Matt, don't expect me to be impressed with your purchase! Spending grocery money on almost a *year's* supply of laundry detergent? But foregoing essentials like milk, bread and eggs? That's *not* smart thinking! Have you even a single dollar left to do your laundry?" Pausing for a nanosecond, he jumped in.

"Mum! You worry too much! *You* taught me how to buy good deals. How could I resist? I've *never ever* seen soap at such a good price. There was a limit—so naturally I complied. Carrying four huge bottles was pretty heavy, especially since I had to walk three blocks home. Still, only stopped to rest a few times." Pride wafted through the phone line.

"My turn, Matt! Your weekly budget is meant for food essentials and washing clothes, before loading up on good deals. How can you not get that?"

"Yah, I guess. Still, not taking any bottles back—my money, my choice! Promise next week I'll save money for laundry. Might still have a few clean clothes left. I'll be okay without milk too. Gotta go find space for all these bottles." Then giggling at his dilemma, "Don't know where though. Bye."

Familiar waves of tension undulated below my skin. "Night, Matt. I love you."

Motherly layers of complexity are not easy to define and separate. Intellectually I've learned not to feel like a hypocrite, despite extended epic clashes of personal values with life's realities. Watching Matt's strong beginnings erode and tides of potential wash away before my eyes initially left me shattered.

My outer public shell had been broken and my heart mirrored it well. I embarked on a deeply contemplative journey—an emotional archaeological dig. Long and short stints of arduous sifting were followed by periods of exhaustion and inertia. Such a worthwhile journey couldn't be rushed.

The crux of my anguish surfaced. How could I be culpable if I had done my best as a fallible human being? My head pleaded *not guilty*. My heart was a harder sell.

After deep soul searching, enlightenment awaited. My unique shortcomings, good intentions and human frailties are fused by lifelong commitment and unwavering love. The verdict? I'm flawed, not a fraud. The warrior angel analogy upheld under scrutiny. My spirit stirred. Deep within, plumes of stale energy were released. Muscle memory reminded weathered wings how to flutter and hover with ease in the viscous air of life.

With gobs of emotional glue I reconfigured my broken vision of hopes, dreams and possibilities. The vision remains, albeit reconfigured, fractured into large chunks and small shards. Assessing, integrating and valuing every misaligned piece is natural, honest and uniquely mine. Each element of the meditative process contributed to the development of my emotional Picasso. It doesn't matter if anyone else understands it, because I do.

The excavation unearthed a treasure—a crystal of truth, that fear and guilt long denied me. I am *not* in control of how my son's life unfolds.

That truth also applies to our daughter. The difference is Kate has the capacity to recognize her missteps and recalibrate her compass. That precious gift eludes Matt—a gift most take for granted.

Shedding misguided guilt about somehow failing my son has been freeing. Absorbing the truth drop by drop has helped nourish withering advocacy roots. Occasionally wisps of guilt waft by, inviting me to revisit shortcomings and regrets. With practice, I've learned to shoo them away.

Until my last breath, I will be a staunch advocate for my son. My ongoing challenge is to respect that Matt's at the helm, steering his life's course. Mother doesn't always know best.

Matt is creating *his* own Picasso. And it's taking shape. Ultimately the direction and design rests with him. All our family can do is seek to understand his creation. And isn't that the way with all art—designed by the artist and open to interpretation by all?

Chapter 26: Interwoven Threads

Stepping back is required to embrace the whole. Threads of warp and woof created this distinctive, imperfect fabric of my adulthood and motherhood. Predominantly subtle patterns intersect with daring splashes of boldness. Career and personal life coalesced into one, as life stranded threads in unimaginable ways.

A diverse and rewarding career path became interlaced with my life as the mother of a vulnerable son with challenges. All the elements of drama are inextricably interwoven. I've basked in periods of harmony when the alignment of warp and woof was impeccable. Frequent times of high tension stretched taut threads to the breaking point. During rough patches of inevitable tangled messes, the focus was on basic survival. Honing knotting skills was critical. Loose threads quickly unravelled. Gaping holes needed mending, delicately integrating lost stitches back into the whole—permanent reminders of battle fatigue, skirmishes and resilience. Countless threads created the invisible garment that cloaks and defines me.

As a young adult in the throes of university exams, initial threads of opportunity were dropped unexpectedly at my feet. A procrastinator at heart, I'd deferred applying for an obscurely written child-care counsellor position—too long. My job application arrived after the position was filled. The "hospital school" director informed me by letter, closing in an unusual fashion—with an enticing job offer. It was a pilot project position, teaching preschoolers with significant disabilities. Didn't matter that I lacked teaching qualifications or experience. All children in the facility were wards of the government and bore a wide range of diagnoses, including physical and intellectual disabilities. With a pending marriage and no job, I jumped into the abyss. This first dip into the world of disability was as a fresh university graduate in 1971. My lifelong career in human services began in the arena of institutionalization, not inclusion.

The enlightened facility director wanted stimulation for children in the preschool unit. Prior to creating my position, mobile youngsters spent their days wandering in their cavernous, sterile unit, with its beige cinder-block walls. Devoid of decor, the only rays of sunshine came from windows much too high to look out. Wrapped in despondency, this locked unit was identified only as C Unit. Children with significant mobility challenges frequently stared at dust bunnies under heat registers while resting on mats, waiting. Waiting for the day's highlights—meals, shift changes and bedtime.

I worked one-on-one with a few select children. Without a curriculum, I focused on natural learning opportunities, individualizing my approach for each child. During lunch in the cafeteria, teachers sighed over misbehaving children who were sometimes sent to detention rooms. Brimming with elation, I frequently shared breakthrough moments from the morning.

"Omigod, Marilyn recognized herself in the mirror. She touched her own nose and was mesmerized to see her counterpart do the same." Or "Billy learned to turn the doorknob today. Been working on it for weeks."

I witnessed major strides in learning and became more adept at recognizing potential, hidden under the weight of disability and low expectations. My workplace was a facility that I left every weekday to go home. That same facility, with its locked units, was deemed home for vulnerable children in the care of government staff, not families. In my third year of work I occasionally picked up my preschool students on weekends, taking them on outings to my parents' home so they could experience a change of environment. It was a different time.

Shielding myself from a broken marriage, I risked leaving the job and my hometown of Saint John. Determined to regain stability and stretch my capacity for self-reliance, I returned to Halifax. It held fond university memories and the prospect of a few friends. Without the security of a job, I agreed to be a stranger's roommate, based solely on the recommendation of a mutual acquaintance, someone from our parents' generation. Jumping this chasm of uncertainty opened a new chapter where independence and maturity awaited.

While looking for work, I enrolled in a six-week women's karate class, solely as an exercise program. Not having an athletic bone in my body, it was an awkward fit. The imprint of a failed marriage was not going to plague me, so I promised myself never to quit karate when I felt like "a loser." Struggling through initial periods of self-doubt nurtured personal capacity and opened my eyes.

Perseverance and effort helped me appreciate the fluid, ongoing balance of mind, body, and spirit inherent in this ancient art. Those eternal conflicts resonated deeply as part of all human struggle. What started as a six-week course evolved into over four decades of traditional karate training. This discipline helped engrave invaluable life lessons—be keenly aware, stand up for what one believes in, stay rooted, know when and how to block, deflect, walk away and attack.

My hiatus from the work world lasted a few unsettling months. Fortunately, I was hired by the City of Halifax, initially as a social assistance worker. My career flourished as did my self-confidence, working under visionary program managers. Through their efforts, our social service team experienced an intimate staff development workshop with internationally renowned scholar and activist in the field of developmental disabilities, Dr. Wolf Wolfensberger. He founded the Principle of Normalization, which promoted the inclusion of people with developmental disabilities in ordinary life. That workshop implanted seeds that would be seminal throughout my career. I routinely witnessed the impacts of marginalization and discrimination on devalued citizens. I became driven to stand up. Social justice roots were taking hold.

My human services roles evolved into supervisory responsibility for two program areas, social assistance and a homemaker program for the elderly and disabled. More responsibility was added in the late 1970s—the Supervised Apartment Program. It was an exciting foray into relatively uncharted territory, deinstitutionalization of long-term residents in a mental facility. This initiative was strongly influenced by Dr. Wolfensberger's work. Like my initial job with young children, the focus was on one person at a time. Bogged down by

244

institutional resistance, the work required strategic planning to successfully shepherd people across the marsh.

This new project married aspects of my work across all three programs and became a passion for me. Many candidates had lived in the institution for decades, because of mental health challenges, family breakdown, etc. One woman, Dahlia, was institutionalized at age 12 and released at 52. Return to the community was only possible because of her cousin's loving advocacy and support. Institutional staff tried sabotaging the discharge, stressing risks and warning Dahlia she'd be back. She focused on the prize, seized the opportunity and her life! Dahlia was a wedding guest at my second marriage, to Neil. Life was well balanced as I soared high over smooth waters.

I'd accrued a wealth of program experience with social assistance, as well as supporting the elderly and disabled, but lacked professional qualifications. In the late 1970s, I wielded power over the lives of vulnerable people, granting approval for access to services and disbursement of municipal funds, directly impacting their quality of life. Although I craved philosophy and theory to complement my experience, I was not in a position to quit my job. Opportunity knocked when Dalhousie University's Maritime School of Social Work introduced a Bachelor of Social Work program. To encourage candidates such as myself, the program offered evening classes and credits for significant field experience.

In my first year of marriage, I worked full time, carried a full-time university load and allotted four hours for sleep each night. Neil provided ongoing support and encouragement. When graduation was on the horizon, Alberta government officials approached our social work class to recruit candidates. Their authority was limited to hiring for frontline Child Welfare positions. Knowing you sometimes need to create a wedge to squeak in, I identified that my goal was another supervisory position, noting transferable skills. My clarity nudged the recruiters, who then got approval to conduct a preliminary interview. Their endorsement resulted in a plane ticket for an interview in Edmonton. Daring to advocate for myself propelled our Edmonton move, from pipe dream to reality.

Working in Child Welfare for two years was highly educational, stressful and carried after-hours responsibilities. On the home front, Neil and I had moved into his family home to care for his father— unexpectedly widowed, with multiple serious health conditions, including cancer, emphysema and dementia. My first pregnancy added to the dynamics. I yearned for alignment of work and home life.

Change was in the air. After my maternity leave with Matthew, I resigned to become a Home Care social worker on a pilot project with a cross-disciplinary team. Innovation and teamwork supported frail, elderly individuals to remain at home longer, nurturing informal neighbourhood support as needed. Again, I was fortunate to work under the guidance of a progressive manager and with creative, committed colleagues. Life was good, except for niggling concerns that Matthew's early milestones were somewhat delayed. At work, political winds shifted, our beloved leader left and program uncertainty mounted. I started looking for new options.

My blend of professional and personal experience with vulnerable populations helped bolster my resume. My new position as social work coordinator in an extended care centre meant working with adults of all ages who lived with bodily frailties, dementia and developmental disabilities. There was a specifically designated Young Adult Unit, which housed young people, many of whom were institutionalized after a traumatic injury. Every resident was designated as needing a full-time care environment. I wasn't so convinced. Regimentation of routines and processes didn't align with my penchant for flexibility and individualized approaches. The grating increased, like shifting tectonic plates.

I recall being asked to attend a meeting between a nursing supervisor and an upset family. They wanted minor adjustments in the approach to their elderly father's care. Repeatedly citing policy and practice restrictions, the supervisor plopped the thick administrative binder on her desk. Firmly entrenched, she asked if they'd like to read any specific policies. My attempts to reason and bridge the divide were in vain—she'd have none of it. Beaten down by the nurse's broken record, the dejected couple left, with shoulders slumped and eyes cast downward.

"They just don't get it," the supervisor said, shaking her head and returning her policy bible to its drawer. It was useless to say that my perspective varied drastically.

I stood and sighed "Time for me to go." There was no turning back. The search was on to find work that aligned with my values, focusing on caring versus being *in care*.

My interview went well with an Alberta government program that became rebranded as Persons with Developmental Disabilities (PDD). Within hours, the regional manager called and offered me the new position of Supervisor, Client Services Coordination. I followed a wise friend's suggestion and requested a follow-up interview. That extra step would give me full control—a chance to understand the position better and assess how well the program's philosophy and values aligned with my own.

Eager to fill the position, the manager hastily rearranged his schedule to squeeze me in. He advised that the human resources representative would phone me shortly with details of the offer. That way he'd have the paperwork ready to sign when we met. During discussions with the representative she discovered an error in the posting of the salary range. Accepting this job would mean no initial salary increase and a shorter vacation allotment—too big a leap.

The follow-up interview was set for early the next morning and I'd already booked the day off. In all good conscience I needed to inform the enthusiastic manager in person. I would decline the job offer.

"You sure?" Neil pressed as I donned my coat.

"Sadly, yes. If they'd posted the correct salary scale I wouldn't even have applied. And now here I am, ready to waste this busy man's time and a precious vacation day. I'll be back shortly." I kissed him on the cheek and left.

Upon returning home, I tossed my hat into the air and shouted, "Just accepted a new job! Oh hon, I loved the program's philosophy, approach and focus on individual needs."

Neil gave a sly smile. "Somehow, not really surprised. When do you start?"

My new career grounded me. It restored equilibrium of personal and professional philosophies. And so began a rewarding and educational 19-year career focused on the goal of supporting adults with developmental disabilities to live as citizens in their communities. I accepted the initial position while having no idea that our son would eventually fall under the program's mandate. Matthew was only seven and his primary diagnosis was still two years away. Parental concerns continued to mount over our son's development, which lagged behind all classmates.

Settling into my position I began to recognize the importance of tailoring the match between families and the designated coordinator. One determined coordinator, Blossom, stood out as being overly confident in her skills and rigid in her views. She made no bones about it: the team didn't need a supervisor, especially someone from the outside. She had no patience for families she deemed as overindulging sons and daughters who "just needed a firm hand." It had a familiar ring to it. Matt was not yet a teenager, but her stance gave me a glimpse into what could await if we sought services in adulthood.

One day Blossom coldly asked me to join her in the boardroom for a case conference, at the family's request. When I introduced myself, the parents lifted their heads. All I saw was pain, anguish and concerns. They showed courage by daring to ask for supervisory input. I used diplomacy to mediate. Not wholeheartedly endorsing the coordinator's narrow perspective was considered betrayal. Blossom made that clear later, as she stormed down the hall

248

muttering. However, the family gained leverage and left with a bit of hope. No government wall was erected—at least on that day.

Realistically, caseload size and worker availability influenced assignment more than ensuring a good match—a common sad theme across government programs. Inherent complexities and limitations in the system created hurdles to meeting the goals of the government and the people it served.

After a few months in the position, I was privileged to watch the Provincial PDD Director, Norm McLeod, walk the talk of inclusion. Norm unexpectedly joined a late-day case conference with a mother and her advocate from the Alberta Association for Community Living (AACL). Collectively the trio made a convincing case for adopting a more flexible approach to policy implementation. It was my first experience with families using advocates to help challenge the system into embracing individualized approaches. This early introduction to the power of advocacy became enmeshed in almost two decades of government work in the field of services to adults with disabilities.

Matthew clearly qualified for paid support through the broader Children's Services disability mandate. Yet I shrugged off everyone's suggestions to apply. I couldn't reconcile that program's focus on addressing deficits, with my focus on fostering capacity. When Matt was in his mid-teens, exhaustion triumphed over dread. Accessing in-home support allowed me to resume neglected karate training. Those two evenings weekly helped keep a grip on my sanity. I couldn't help but wonder if attending to my needs might take my eyes off the ball and inadvertently invite a slide into *clienthood*. But if I neglected my own mental health….

After a few years in the Edmonton regional office, I was approached about a lateral transfer, to work on a provincial project. Honoured, I worked on a cross-ministry committee with the goal of promoting inclusion. As a secondary player representing PDD, the experience educated me on the power of advocacy, entrenchment, allies and strategic negotiation. Around boardroom tables I witnessed veteran strategists clash. Embers of discontent were fanned and erupted into flames, as program perspectives varied. I was totally mesmerized by everyone's skills. Flying close to the fire, I felt the heat without getting my wings singed. At the end of the allotted term, I was asked to stay, moving into a provincial policy position.

Philosophically and programmatically focusing on inclusion was under the inspired leadership of Norm McLeod and his team of equally enlightened directors. I was amazed at their collective encouragement to challenge the status quo. Parental perspectives and those of inclusion advocates were actively sought and highly valued in the provincial arena.

Early in my orientation to the world of provincial policy I recall a last-minute request from Norm to represent him at a cross-ministry meeting. I was floored.

"What? But I'm not apprised of all the issues and unsure what stance you'd like me to take."

Norm gave his sweet, reassuring smile. "Be guided by where the discussions lead. You're well grounded in our program philosophy and principles. And as a mum of someone who in adulthood may well qualify for program support, trust your gut. Whatever you say will work for me. Best get moving—your meeting starts in a half hour."

Stunned and honoured, he handed me the agenda and rushed off to another pressing meeting. Norm's trust and encouragement was like being handed a *talking stick*, with the power to be heard and influence.

For many years I served as Alberta's program policy manager, serving adults with developmental disabilities. Throughout government, official program names change as government priorities shift and programs shuffle under different ministerial umbrellas.

During my tenure, I always walked a tightrope seeking balance. Fostering a policy framework and practices that supported inclusion had its challenges. Progressive forces battled patronization from the old guard within bureaucratic and political arenas, as well as some entrenched community sectors. Program dynamics were blended in a larger provincial vessel with jurisdictional, historical and political considerations galore.

Provincial consultation with individuals and families, followed by negotiated wording with the service sector, produced our program's Principles for Determining Individual Support Needs. The foundation principle is timeless in its relevance: *Individuals, with the assistance of families and friends, are the primary source for identifying what is best for themselves and what kind of support they require.*

Supplementary principles were created to guide program-funded supports, whether provided through agencies or family-managed services. I framed this pivotal document, forever cherishing its bold truths. In theory, implementation was a given, but pushback was strong.

Well before Matt reached adulthood, I chaired a PDD provincial committee that developed the Abuse Prevention and Reporting (APR) Protocol. The emphasis was on awareness, education and collaboration, rather than a punitive approach to addressing non-criminal concerns. The innovative protocol, which applied to all PDD-funded arrangements, earned a prestigious Premier's Award of Excellence.

Later, the protocol was affected by new broad-based legislation, the Protection for Persons in Care Act (PPC Act). The legislation took a hardline institutional approach, applying to a wide array of designated care facilities, such as extended care centres, hospitals and institutions identified under other legislative acts. As with all legislation there's always room for interpretation. PDD recognized that it would not go untouched. After all, it still funded facilities where eligibility criteria, program standards and round-the-clock staffing ruled. This included formal institutions and group homes.

PDD wanted its protocol, instead of legislation to address concerns in typical community living settings, such as apartments and private dwellings. These were people's homes, not institutions. I was assigned the lead PDD role in navigating clarity of the legislative scope, with the goal of minimizing impact on our program. Both PDD and PPC representatives met with our mutual legal counsel to debate and interpret the Act's scope. PDD believed that "designated facilities" should be readily recognizable to common citizens, applying normative community standards.

Intrigued, the lawyer asked probing questions and I explained how the APR protocol would be applied to typical community settings. He was fully engaged and followed the logic. Staff spearheading the new PPC Act immediately countered, pressing for sweeping coverage of all PDD-funded situations. They stressed that a legislative approach would eliminate stakeholder confusion, ensure nobody was missed and protect the minister from any associated risk. Scepticism crept into the room and shooed common sense out the door.

A sledgehammer approach now applied to all allegations involving people received PDD funding, regardless of the setting. I lay bloodied on the bureaucratic battlefield with gaping wounds. The applauded APR protocol slowly began to bleed out. As a mother, I was later reminded that policy and interdepartmental roles didn't inoculate me from the wrath of a system scorned. I unintentionally unleashed flames of PPC institutional processes—a spark on a dry bale of hay.

Prior to that personal nightmare, PDD's incredible leader had retired, government ministries were reconfigured and our program was being course corrected. There were countless adjustments in approaches and expectations that ran counter to our program's mission, vision and values. For years I experienced great synchronicity of personal and professional values. It was easy to pour heart and soul into work I believed in. I recall one official saying "The Norm McLeod era is over." Oh boy, did we know it!

Work was now like a Rubik's cube with a new twist provided daily. Still serving as provincial policy manager, documents that I supposedly played a role in developing looked foreign. Unable to follow PDD program logic and decipher its code left me looking and feeling inept. Was I losing my mind? Almost 20 years of satisfying work rapidly eroded and I was in quicksand.

Personal risks were too grave to attempt carrying on for a final year, when I'd be eligible for an unreduced pension. Each day tightened threads around my growing stress ball. Another wrap or two could be fatal, both physically and emotionally. With a rapidly withering soul, I explored meaningful career transfers. I was desperate to avoid leaving a much-loved career with a bitter taste. Incredibly, an intriguing opportunity arose for a lateral transfer back to the regional PDD office. I gladly left the Rubik's cube behind.

Thankfully this was a period of stability on the Matt front. He'd moved to an apartment close by, relying on family support and auditing the Radio and Television Arts program at the Northern Alberta Institute of Technology (NAIT).

In my final year until retirement I supervised an innovative regional PDD pilot project. It focused on assessing quality of life for people receiving services. The scope of the work was manageable, readily achievable and made good sense. I regained equilibrium, worked within a familiar operational framework and was shielded from the "puzzle palace" madness.

I wanted my retirement to be celebrated by a simple open house for coffee and cake on my last day of work. I was honoured that many people I'd worked with over the years attended, from both the community and government sectors. Everyone, including me, was impressed with Matt who employed his emerging expertise with NAIT camera equipment to film the speeches. Surprisingly, the PPC director attended and gave me a token gift with the PPC logo on it.

As we gathered up the boxes of mementos, gifts and cards, Matt noticed the PPC gift remaining on my desk. "Almost forgot something. Take this too Mum?"

"Nope, it stays. Maybe someone else will have a use for it."

About six months after my government farewell, I was lured out of retirement by Cindy, a former colleague. She'd left the confines of government, in favour of community advocacy. The regional PDD pilot program was ready to launch into the community, under the wings of Gateway Association for Community Living. I was hooked by Cindy's passion, leadership style and nature of the work. Working part-time, with diverse, spirited and committed colleagues was both meaningful and dare I say fun.

At Gateway I felt understood and unconditionally supported during good times and bad times with Matt, while highly respected for my values and contributions. The Gateway experience was my swan song. Reminiscing about the fabric of my life's work, I am grateful for the many years of personal and professional alignment. Those memories keep me cozy, wrapped in my densely woven retirement cloak. No regrets.

Courage and Endurance

Chapter 27: Time to Be Brave

With voices coated in apprehension, we sang happy birthday. Our eldest had turned 18, denoting adulthood in Alberta. When the server approached at our celebratory lunch, Matt's smile almost swallowed his face.

"We're ready to order. I'm the birthday boy—no, birthday man actually. And since I turned 18 today, I'll have a beer with my food. I've got my ID ready 'cause I know you need to check it. Bet some people try to fool you, but not me. Yah, it'll be my first beer ever." It went down smoothly, so he ordered a second.

Striving to be cool was extremely important to our son, as for most young people. When Matt tried something new, he typically immersed himself in the experience, until the newness wore off. Experimentation with drinking was no exception.

Shortly after Matt's birthday, he moved to a small town, becoming an Olds College student. He was enrolled in a specialized transitional vocational program for young adults. On a weekend visit home, Matt and a friend went bar hopping Friday night. They drank well past the point of oblivion. After midnight, Matt recognized his incapacity to get himself safely home, so called his faithful cousin from the bar phone.

"Hello…Martin? S'Matt! Sorry ta bother ya but I'm kinda, well not kinda…I'm totally drunk, plastered, 'nebriated, shit-faced or whatever else ya wanna call it. Money's gone so no cab home. And bus drivers can't let drunk people on. Even if I convinced a driver, couldn't walk the final few blocks home...Martin? Martin you still there?"

"Yah I'm here, still trying to wake up. Matt, tell me where you are. I'll drive you home."

"Thanks, Cuz. You're the best. Please call my parents too; bartender wants me to get off the phone. Oh boy, they'll be pissed—just like me, but in a different way. Know what I mean?"

"Sure do, I'll call them. Be waiting for me outside in 15 minutes."

Martin left his warm bed to retrieve Matt and delivered him home. Leaning heavily on Martin who propped him up, Matt staggered up the sidewalk and grasped our front porch railing.

"Whoa, didn't think these stairs were so steep," he said as he clutched the railing. With great effort and guidance, he pulled himself up the five stairs. Miraculously the railing remained bolted to the porch.

"Hi Mum, Dad. Sorry, sorry for you know…had to call Martin. Couldn't have made it home otherwise."

Neil and Martin exchanged looks and silently prepared for the tricky exchange. It was as fluid as a high-calibre ice dancing routine. Martin slipped out from under Matt's weight, slightly tipping Matt's balance to the other side, where Neil assumed full control.

A surprised, bleary-eyed Matt said, "Huh…well that was easy. Gotta get to bed, but bathroom first." Unimpressed, but glued to his side for safety purposes Neil escorted him to both destinations. Thank God it was the weekend so we could sleep in. Theoretically at least.

Both kids' bedrooms were upstairs and the sole bathroom was downstairs, with a hairpin turn on the stairwell. As dawn reared its head, the aftermath of drunkenness took control. Violently ill and unable to stand up, Matt bellowed for help, waking everyone up, again. He was totally incapacitated, so the unpleasantness and messy loads of laundry were left for me. "Sorry, Mum" just didn't cut it.

Everybody was in a foul mood except for Matt. He moaned and groaned, in self-pity. He didn't grasp why there was a shortage of sympathy.

"Wasn't like I planned to get sick. Ohhh, I feel awful. Can you get me more ginger ale and crackers? Maybe it'll stay down this time." The link between actions and natural consequences was lost on Matt.

He only dragged himself from bed to use the bathroom. Our young adult was fully in the clutches of a horrific hangover. By Sunday lunchtime his sickness had abated enough to keep a small bowl of soup down. The lament about feeling awful continued and our patience ran thin. Everyone nipped at each other like hungry snapping turtles.

On Sunday evening, with brown bags in his backpack and a greenish hue to his face, we guided Matt onto the Greyhound bus for his trip back to college. A woman I knew happened to be catching the same bus. Being the mother of young men herself, she recognized Matt's fragility and kindly offered to keep a watchful eye over him. He made it back to his dorm safely and without getting sick. I took that as a glimmer of hope at the end of a lost weekend. Dark days and darker nights were still ahead.

Matt missed classes Monday and Tuesday, as he was still having problems retaining food and drink. I attributed this to ingesting too much, too quickly. The next morning, I visited Matt while en route to a conference in Calgary. He looked pasty and sapped of energy. He barely talked over lunch and sparsely sampled his soup. While his discomfort pulled at my heartstrings, this was a life lesson he'd learn the hard way. I returned him to his dorm with ample ginger ale and crackers—the foundation for a speedy recovery.

It didn't help. Matt called my hotel room late Wednesday evening. "Mum, I'm still really sick. I even walked to the hospital emergency. They said I'm really dehydrated and wanted to rehydrate me. But they needed to do it intravenously. You know how I am."

"Oh Matt, I know needles terrify you. Were you brave enough to handle it?"

"Nah, it was way too scary. The nurse said she could use a smaller needle, a *butterfly needle* I think. But I just couldn't. So I walked back home. I think teachers are getting mad at me for not goin' to any classes. But I'm still too sick."

"Sweetheart, getting rehydrated is important. I'm hoping you go back tomorrow and specifically ask for the butterfly needle. It'll be worth it; trust me. Think about it?"

"I'll try."

"In the morning I'll call the college, explain and ask your program coordinator to check on you. Get some sleep now. Night!"

I became worried as Thursday evening wore on. I'd not heard from Matt. Finally he called close to midnight. Early in the evening his concerned program coordinator drove him back to the hospital. By then he was desperate for relief. His words were scarcely audible. Sheer exhaustion had stretched his voice as thin as a mist.

"Did it, Mum. Nurse used a butterfly needle. Took two, no three full bags to rehydrate me—maybe more. Can't remember I'm so tired. They said I should feel better real quick. Night."

After hanging up, I decided that Matt had suffered enough. I'd leave the conference early the next day, pick him up and nurse him back to health at home.

On Friday morning I couldn't contact Matt or his program coordinator to share my plans. Panic started to take hold. Neil tried reaching somebody at the college who could update us. Meanwhile I hit the highway.

Eventually Neil learned that Matt's program coordinator escorted Matt back to the hospital on Friday morning. His pounding headache had become incapacitating. The doctor recommended a CAT scan but the local hospital lacked the equipment. So the coordinator kindly escorted him to the nearest city hospital in Red Deer. That's where I caught up with him. Fortunately, the doctor was in the room when I arrived. A look of relief washed across Matthew's face when he saw me.

"Here's my mum now. How'd you find me? The doctor was starting to tell me about tests they did."

"You're Matthew's mother?" I nodded, seeking answers with my eyes. "Well the CAT scan shows that Matthew has a subdural hematoma. We need to transfer him right away to a major hospital that can deal with this. I'll arrange to have him transported to Calgary."

"Doctor, we live in Edmonton so would like him transferred there. I'm heading home right away and can drive him directly to the designated hospital."

"Transferring him to an Edmonton hospital is no problem. It'll be good to have family available. However, you driving him is not an option. He'll be transported by ambulance, immediately. If you wait a few minutes at the desk, the nurse will tell you which hospital he's going to." Then the porter arrived.

I numbly walked with them to the ambulance bay. As Matt's stretcher was being secured, I offered words of reassurance. "I'll be right behind you. If your driver speeds, I will too. Betcha the police wouldn't give me a ticket!" I blew him a kiss and the ambulance doors slammed shut.

My pasted smile disappeared as they sped away with lights flashing and sirens screaming. The gravity of the situation started to hit home. The doctor's diagnosis was an ominous jumble of words. I needed my husband.

Hearing Neil's voice on the phone, my protective shield fell, exposing raw fear. Leaning against a wall outside the emergency department I managed to blubber my way through. Endless tears washed my face clean. I didn't care who saw me.

"Oh, hon, I'm so scared. I wish you were here; you'd have understood all the medical jargon. Can't remember what the doctor called it; something like *subduratoma*."

"What? Did you say *subdural hematoma*?" There was no mistaking the lead weight in Neil's voice.

"Yes. Dear God, what does that mean?" His initial silence—like the flash from a distant lightning bolt—conveyed a powerful message. I sensed that our world was about to reverberate.

"Time for talking later. I'll be waiting for Matt when the ambulance arrives. Get here as fast as you can. Drive safe though; I'll be at his side. Susan…we will get through this."

A thorough assessment revealed that Matt needed surgery, performing what the medical profession calls a mini-crani. The surgery required drilling a hole in Matt's skull to release pressure on his brain. The surgeon told us that he would temporarily remove a piece of Matt's skull, the size of a two-dollar Canadian coin, a toonie.

The doctor explained: "This is what is called a contre-coup head injury. It's sustained when a severe blow causes the brain to bounce in its cerebral fluid from one side of the skull to the other and back again. In your son's case, the associated bleeding caused the pressure that we'll alleviate through the mini-crani surgery." This time I was held up by Neil's warm embrace, not a cold hospital wall.

Matt returned from surgery, bald with a vulgar plug in his skull, adorned by 17 silver staples. Once past the shock, my eyes didn't need to look. That first post-surgery glance had done its work. With the stroke of a master craftsman's blowtorch the scorched image was vividly etched into my mind.

Still grappling with the cause of such a head injury, we repeatedly sought answers. "Matt did you fall or did someone hit you? Do you remember anything bad happening?" He hadn't recalled any such event, so the mystery continued.

For days I sat by his hospital bed while our son slept, except for short intervals. Intuitively rubbing my chest, I tried to caress my aching heart. This self-soothing gesture helped me feign calmness and bravery when he was awake.

After a few days a nurse announced. "Okay, Matt let's get you up and your legs moving." She helped him sit up and get stable. "This walker will help give you some balance."

Turning to stretch my neck for a moment, I heard "No, no, no young man! You need to let me lock the wheels first and show you how to drive it." Smiling, she teased: "You don't want me to get in any trouble now, do you?" Matt had become a favourite with nurses, being extremely polite and grateful for all of their help.

That first day, with the walker, we took frequent mini-strolls. We walked as far as two doors down the hall before fatigue demanded a rest. Within a half hour, Matt was ready to get back at it. The next day, after successfully reaching three doorways, Matt was determined to ditch the walker. He'd definitely inherited his mother's tendency to be naïvely optimistic about how easy something would be.

"Mum, I need to walk farther every day, so let's get started. Been walking since I was little, so my brain should remember pretty quick." Nurses and I exchanged looks of caution while not wanting to dampen his enthusiasm to regain basic skills.

"Okay, but there are ground rules. Walk close to the wall so you can grab the wall railing if you need it. I'll stay beside you in case you need extra support. And, we'll head back to the room when I notice that you're starting to get tired."

"Fine. Let's go."

Initially, without the walker, we didn't get far. Our son doggedly kept trying, despite poor balance and energy levels that plummeted without warning. While stamina was in short supply, his determination was infinite.

After a short rest I'd hear: "Okay Mum, I'm ready. Let's try going one door farther. I wanna get home. The doctor says not until I can walk past four doors in the hall, each and every time." The hard work paid off within a few days.

Waiting at the elevator after his release, our eldest looked deep in my eyes. "Mum, I don't think I've ever been so brave in my life."

"Same here. Now let's go home." Elevator doors opened and we began the next step of his recovery, from home.

Matt's balance issues were improving, but not resolved. I fretted at the prospect of sleeping in his upstairs bedroom, navigating the hairpin turn. Matt's pleas prevailed and I lived with my fear, hovering whenever he climbed the stairs. It helped to rest comfortably in his own bed, surrounded by his belongings and nurtured by his loving cat, Scooter.

The first evening Matt was home Kate knocked on his bedroom door then entered. "Matt, remember, I'm across the hall so if you need anything, just holler. Bet you thought you'd never hear me say that! Until you're all better I'll let you get away with it. Now have a good sleep—you too, Scooter!" Hearing his name, the devoted cat poked his head from under the blanket.

Matt showed us that he, like everyone else, has the capacity to face challenges beyond what one can imagine. Our family's mettle was tested. Individual and family networks wrapped us in wide wings of loving support. People assisted in countless direct and indirect ways that will never be forgotten.

Supportive colleagues shared my workload, allowing me to work reduced hours. Arriving home around noon, I'd soon hear Matt starting to stir from his sleep.

"Okay Matt, what adventure should we go on this afternoon?" Daily outings helped break the boredom of being housebound.

We focused on whatever interested him. That included riding on an articulating bus, checking out active construction sites (always of intense interest) and going to favourite bustling spots downtown. We were on the move and that was all that mattered.

Initially, Matt wore a baseball cap to hide the disturbing surgery site, yet it rarely stayed on for long. I learned to ignore the stares of strangers that went unnoticed by Matt.

One day as we closed the front door Matt said: "Think you forgot my ball cap."

His innocent comment caught me off guard. Truth be told, the ball cap issue was mine, not his. Time to release control.

"I can nab it, but only if you want to wear it."

"Nope. Let's get going, Mum. I really want to show you where…" And off we went.

Despite the inevitability of plummeting energy and altered balance, we pushed the envelope by staying out a little longer each time. Enhancing his stamina resulted in moments of critical decision-making. One moment he was fine and within seconds his legs would start to buckle.

"Okay, Matt. That's our cue to stop, now. Your choice—I can help you to the bench on the corner, before running to bring the car around, or we can hail a taxi to drive us to the car."

"Mum, that's not fair for the driver—our car's not far away so he'd only get a little money. Just take my arm and I'll wait for you on the bench." I ran to the car, helped him in and we headed home to share our adventures. Every small stride was a win.

The doctor was pleased with Matt's progress. When it was time for the staples to be removed, every muscle in my body convulsed. Unable to look, I turned away, swaying and hugging myself.

"All done," the doctor announced. "Good job holding still, Matt. Your head is healing nicely. You'll always have a big scar to remind you of this rough patch. You and your family have been working hard to get your stability back and it shows. Still have a long way to go though; maybe up to a year." Looking directly at Neil and me he cautioned, "Even then, it might only be a partial recovery. There's just no guarantee."

The prospect struck terror in our hearts. To stack the odds in Matt's favour, we engaged therapists in reiki therapy, energy flow and therapeutic massage.

When Matt felt brave enough, his trusted barber ever so carefully cut his hair, offering reassurances as he gingerly snipped near the surgery site. The haircut was a major accomplishment. The focus on the positive paid off and within six weeks, Matt was deemed recovered enough for a trial return to college.

We tentatively solved the mystery of what happened, bit by bit. Minimally, the pieces assembled in a way that made sense, to the doctor and us. Initially, Matt was likely battling alcohol poisoning, which could account for the prolonged poor recovery from his drinking binge. The final puzzle piece was found when Matt returned to college.

Neil and I had stopped to thank the program coordinator for her wonderful support. While discussing the mystery of it all, she recalled something important.

"I didn't think about it at the time but that Thursday evening when I drove Matt to the Olds hospital, he misjudged the passenger door opening. He dropped his whole body weight when getting in and hit his head on the car doorframe. The force of it made my stomach turn. Matt cried out in pain and rubbed his head the whole way there."

After sharing this key puzzle piece, the doctor said this explanation totally matched the profile of Matt's head injury. Having a plausible theory gave us some comfort.

264

While physical balance was regained, emotional stability was more elusive—a common issue when someone incurs a head injury. The pressure on Matt's brain was released. What seems to remain is a tangled web of cranky neurons that seek a peaceful place in his psyche. They seem to have found a fairly comfortable nest. However, just like a quiet wasp's nest, unpredictability is a given when poked. Bravery is always on call.

Chapter 28: Systematically Yours

The refrain of an old rock tune resounds in my head. It perfectly captures the essence of government support systems. As Trooper's lyrics say, "she's a three dressed up as a nine." Like the girl in the song, upon closer scrutiny, government's accountability for its rhetoric falls short. Bureaucratic documents are carefully crafted, polished and tightly controlled. Rhythmically the words sound clear, strong and pure. Families seeking support seize the superficial message, prepared to learn unnatural dance steps to participate. They're at a huge disadvantage, lacking the musician's knowledge and sheet music to interpret subtle nuances of wording and intent.

Therein lies the rub. Both dance partners hear the words but interpret them differently. Government and funded agencies lead, while families strive to follow, seeking partnership in a fluid interpretive dance. Power rests with the heavily resourced system, not the family seeking support. As always, it's the little guy's toes that get stepped on. I know—I've been on both sides. My arthritic fingers and toes are a daily reminder that I've stretched every sinew, taken chances and paid a price.

I'm critically aware of inherent restrictions that every public servant faces, no matter how empathetic and dedicated. Unexpectedly, wildcards get played—bureaucratic structural changes, belt tightening or political upheaval. Change is the only constant. As a parent I worked to seize opportunities, loose threads or loopholes— before they morphed or vaporized. Staying current demanded vigilance, time, energy and effort. Sometimes I earned a passing grade and other times failed miserably.

When adulthood arrived for Matt, we supported him to spread his wings and leave the family nest. The opportunity to have his own apartment with ready access to daytime staffing support sounded promising. Still, my gut told me to be wary. After collapsing on the couch from a long, tiring day, I confided in Neil. He'd just picked up the TV remote when I spilled my concerns.

"Hon, I have reservations about Matt's prospective move. The agency's history is so entrenched in segregation and group-home mentality. Their new independent living apartment complex is enticing and well intentioned, but what a huge leap of faith! What if they can't make the transition?" Neil put down the remote and turned to me.

"It's akin to jumping over a campfire...definitely a gamble. But we want Matt to start living the life of a young adult and that means independence—for him and us. And didn't you say more progressive agencies all have long waiting lists?"

"Right on all counts. It'll be a huge stretch for this agency to match their new rhetoric with equally progressive approaches. Okay, let's jump across the flames and hope not to get burned." I squeezed his hand and picked up the remote.

Issues abounded from the get-go. The agency was glued to program-based approaches and practices. What made sense to them didn't support any typical community sniff test. For example the staff person, Beth, answered the office phone with "Rez 12" versus "Hello."

"Oh Susan, it really doesn't mean anything. I'm just so used to saying that in the group homes."

"But this project is intended to be a regular apartment complex, with access to shared support. Referring to it by a residence number entrenches group-home practices—even if it's subconscious." I looked at her, awaiting a response.

"I guess so. Old habits die hard." Beth's voice trailed off, along with her smile.

"Staff know they're calling your office. Couldn't you simply say hello, even adding your name, if you think it's needed?"

"Maybe. I'd have to check." The practice remained and I decided to pick my battles.

Soon the agency proposed the adoption of a laundry schedule. Beth had proactively colour coded a draft weekly schedule—for a building with four tenants.

"We're just trying to accommodate tenant wishes. Kevin likes to do laundry every Friday. Last week he got upset when Matt washed clothes for an unexpected work shift."

"Beth, think about what normally happens in rental situations. An imposed tenant laundry schedule doesn't fit with community norms. I'd recommend support staff facilitating discussion of grievances *only* if tenants unsuccessfully tried working it through independently, as adults. Did Matt's laundry stop Kevin from washing his clothes?"

"No, Kevin still got his laundry done. He only needed to wait a few minutes. We'd just like to avoid the potential for any conflict." A regimented routine would make things clear from the agency perspective, but it was far from being ordinary.

"Learning to resolve conflicts is a basic life skill for every human. You know where we stand on this issue." With slumped shoulders, Beth turned away, ending the conversation. The idea of formalizing a laundry schedule was never raised again.

The agency's weekday office occupied a former basement suite. Tenants were told the agency might also use that space as a training apartment, for residents from group homes. Instituting a segregated day program for group-home residents within this small community apartment complex would make the building stand out, not blend into the neighbourhood.

Beth approached me the first chance she got. "Susan, here's the upside of having a training apartment. The guys who live here could jump in and get some cooking support too." Her smile was forced but her eyes conveyed that she expected resistance.

I took a deep breath, before reinforcing a common theme. "Everything about the idea aligns with institutionalized practices and programs, not typical community living."

Deflated, Beth said, "Got it…you don't want Matt in a group home. That's why he's getting individualized support in an apartment."

"Yes. He and the other men can get your support with cooking skills in their own apartments, right?"

"Of course they can…."

"Exactly. If the agency proceeds with this proposal, it brings group-home ideology to Matt's doorstep and invites it in. That doesn't fly with me."

"Um…well it was just an idea. I kinda get what you're saying. I'll pass your concerns along." Another bone of contention added to the growing pile.

The agency didn't proceed, but not because of me. The regional funding body didn't endorse the proposal, noting that it didn't align with provincial policy. The funder clarified that group home programs could not be incorporated in an independent living setting. Full marks for the regional funder!

Discarding outdated protective practices for a more normative living approach was far harder than the agency expected. Adopting new words was the easy part. Initially tolerated, my relentless scrutiny festered under the agency's skin. I frequently heard "Nobody else seems to mind," or "Really, you're making something out of nothing." Daisy, the friendly project manager, was getting weary of my questioning too. It became apparent that it was our family, not the agency that was deemed out of line.

Before long the agency appointed a site supervisor, Craig. I perceived him as controlling and full of self-importance. With multiple keys of authority jingling from his belt and a puffed-out chest Craig told me that the days of addressing issues with Beth, the on-site staff, were over. He was appointed to oversee operations so everything was to be run by him. He ruled by intimidation. Matt and I were clearly annoyances, both having a penchant for asking why and challenging the rationale.

Anxiety and frustration are core aspects of Matt's disability. Managing anxiety and defusing potential behavioural outbursts requires acknowledgement of his stress, appreciating why he's upset and developing a reasonable plan of action—involving him every step of the way. It doesn't mean pandering to his every wish or excusing inappropriate behaviour. Craig's very presence at the building quickly triggered stress. He adopted a domineering approach to dealing with the tenants in all matters.

One day Matt, who has an incredible eye for detail, noted something awry. "Mum, I noticed that the building's electrical panel is outside. It's on the wall facing the back alley, so anyone could mess with it and leave us in the dark. I think it's dangerous and that makes me nervous."

"Whew, that would be cause for concern. Show me tomorrow and we'll go from there."

"It's unlocked too—I checked. That would definitely violate code. I could call the city and confirm."

"Matt please, there's no need to call the city. I promise to come by in the morning. Leave it until then. Promise?"

"Okay, but it definitely needs to be addressed."

The next day I was shocked to see that Matt was right. I called the supervisor.

Craig exhaled an exasperated sigh. "Hello Mrs. Dunnigan. I presume there's something wrong."

As I started to explain the concern, Craig jumped in. "I'm sure Matt's mistaken. He shouldn't be worried about this kind of stuff anyway. That's our job."

With my inside voice I blasted, "Then do your damn job!" I reminded myself that clarity without a sharp tone would be my best response.

"Craig, I've seen the panel first-hand. Matt's information is accurate and he has every reason to be concerned. I'd like to show you myself, today. How quickly can that happen?" My heart was pounding and I realized I'd been holding my breath. Loosely pursing my lips, I slowly released all the air. It burned with indignation.

Matt peaked from behind his bedroom curtains while I joined the supervisor in the parking lot. Craig swaggered towards the building, stopping short when I pointed out the electrical panel. Instinctively he took a step back, before regaining his authoritative demeanour. Shrugging his shoulders, before walking away, Craig said he'd deal with it. Not a word of thanks or acknowledgement for Matt's diligence.

Property maintenance was sadly neglected, both inside the building and out. The assigned maintenance man, Melvin, had responsibility for other agency-owned buildings. Perpetually grumpy, his trips to the apartment complex were brief and infrequent. The timeworn story was that Melvin had to prioritize his long list and would get to things when he could. It was anything but reassuring and for good reason.

Tenants waited and waited. One issue was a darkened hallway that for weeks had a burned-out light bulb. It was the sole hallway light. One weekend Matt pleaded with me, saying he had lots of experience from home and could easily replace the bare bulb. I saw no harm and he had spares in his apartment. It was an easy fix that didn't require expertise. Supervised by me, Matt stood on a sturdy kitchen chair and restored light to the hallway. The guys all noticed the problem was resolved—staff too. Matt's actions were duly recorded as an infraction. Their rationale cited safety concerns, as well as disrupting Melvin's schedule. Eye rolling increased on both sides.

Hallway upkeep was abysmal. After washing his kitchen floor one day Matt proudly took initiative and mopped the long-neglected hallway floor.

"It was pretty gross, Mum. Had to dump the bucket four times—the first rinse turned the water totally black. Good thing I had lots of Mr. Clean on hand."

The next day it rained while Matt was on a bike ride. Within minutes of returning home Craig knocked at his door. He admonished Matt for leaving residual dirt from his bike wheels in the clean hallway. Addressing outstanding tenant concerns about building maintenance never got any traction. But now Matt's single bike track was an issue.

Feeling targeted, our son panicked whenever Craig was on-site. I often got calls at work. "Matthew, take a breath. He's probably popping into the office for a few minutes. I've not received any complaints. And yes, you can call me back if he knocks on your door."

During winter, the building's overhang deposited a perpetual icy patch on the building's concrete porch. For years, Matt took lead responsibility for de-icing at our family home. He proactively attended to this safety matter without seeking permission. Hearing about the unauthorized action, Craig insisted that Matt not apply sand or de-icer. Only the staff, Beth, who didn't work weekends had access to the de-icer, which was subsequently locked away. The product was well protected, away from the residents it was supposed to protect. It was warped logic. Matt's long-term normative role was being stripped from him. Compliance tightened its screws, digging deep under my skin. Given Matt's lifelong balance issues and risk of slipping, I armed him with a small bag of de-icer to use judiciously, as needed. Facing Craig's wrath was insignificant compared to the risk of Matt getting injured.

Having started his *Lawn Boy* mowing business when he was 10, Matt prided himself on keeping our family's lawn looking well cared for. Our son got increasingly upset when his apartment's lawn stood out as being substantially longer than its community counterparts. Noticeably overgrown before Neil and I went on a two-week vacation, we were told that Melvin would cut the lawn soon. By the time we returned it was a field of dandelions, mostly gone to seed.

"Mum, they keep saying Melvin's busy with other maintenance stuff and will get to it soon. Soon, soon, soon—soon never comes! It's embarrassing to even say I live here." I totally understood. "Please, can I just borrow the lawnmower from home? Lawn's small so I can have it done in 15 minutes. I'll bag it too so there's no mess."

We drove the few blocks home, packed up the mower and I supervised Matt's lawn mowing. As we were packing up Craig stormed around the corner. He was spewing spittle at the audacity of Matt's actions, citing protocols, liability and more. Matt was clearly rattled and I was appalled. We packed up the lawnmower, along with multiple bags of clippings and went for an ice cream.

I subsequently ignited a firestorm by sharing my pent-up frustration with a colleague. Pegi was clear. "Susan, what you've shared clearly warrants looking into as an allegation of abuse."

"Okay. I really just want Craig to step back and show respect. An APR review could be a good thing. When do you think…"

Pegi interrupted me. "I know it definitely wasn't what our program wanted, but PDD regions have recently been notified that any allegations we receive *must* get kicked up to the PPC Act abuse hotline. Non-compliance is deemed a violation of legislation. As you know, legislation trumps policy every time."

"Damn! I don't want a formal PPC Act investigation. Just forget I said anything. The writing's on the wall—time to explore options to this institutional pressure cooker."

"Sorry, Susan. You've shared a number of concerns, which I can't unhear. I could relay the gist of our conversation to the hotline but it's better if you do it yourself." She was right. I made the fateful call.

The powerful PPC machinery, with its legal authority, rumbled in, shaking the ground beneath our feet. Sidelined and stripped of all authority, the APR protocol choked on its dust. A protracted formal investigative process was undertaken, with every concern sliced, diced and adjudicated.

Agency staff closed ranks. Meaningful dialogue seeking further clarification was not part of the equation. Like an inquisition, burning was inevitable. Our family's collective wings of caring were scorched by flame throwers from impenetrable tanks that rolled over the landscape, spewing dust, dirt and debris. We were left to pick through the rubble of dashed hopes and dreams.

Within a few weeks of reporting my concerns, the PDD regional consultant for the agency scheduled a meeting. Al was a nice man, who definitely didn't like conflict.

Perched on the edge of his chair, Al smiled weakly, then folded his hands on his lap and cleared his throat. "It seems both the family and agency have a history of concerns." He stopped to smile awkwardly before continuing. "I appreciate both perspectives, but unfortunately don't really have anything creative to offer."

Al's eyes sought refuge with the project manager, Daisy. Initially eager to work with me on implementation challenges, her enthusiasm sputtered and the spark died out. An intensive course on pathways that support inclusion had pointed her in the right direction, but without agency backing she was spitting into the wind.

Looking straight ahead Daisy got to the point. "We believe our agency has not been a good fit for Matthew."

For a brief moment I was hopeful. "I think everyone acknowledges that we're out of alignment." Maybe her initial vigour for a more inclusive approach was renewed.

"So our agency's decided to give Matt 30 days notice to vacate. We thought it best that you pass the message along to Matt. Al's already aware. We wanted all parties to be represented so everyone is clear." The ensuing silence was deafening.

Rather than extending an olive branch, the agency dropped it. There was no mention of compromise, negotiation and creative problem solving. Not that there was a lot of hope in that option. I had no bargaining chips. Fulfilling the dual role of landlord and service provider, the agency had complete power.

It was the 30 days notice that floored me. Stunned, I looked at Al—my regional colleague who knowingly lured me into the lair. He squirmed. I refused to turn off my high beams.

Sheepishly, glancing down at his papers Al said: "I wish you good luck in finding something more to your liking."

I was far beyond singed by the experience. My psyche was skewered and charbroiled over an open flame, then tarred and feathered by the system.

In the world of disability, community counterfeits routinely masquerade as real. Yet they're cheap knockoffs, a three dressed up as a nine. These settings never hold up to the scrutiny of ordinary living. We were definitely done with this masquerade. The challenge would be to find the real thing...within 30 days.

There was little chance of finding a good, affordable, pet-friendly apartment within close proximity to our family home. We needed an angel of hope. It came in the form of a sign—For Rent.

While this personal drama unfolded, I awkwardly continued my provincial role partnering with senior PPC Act staff on cross-ministerial initiatives. I didn't have much fight left in me, but felt compelled to speak truth to power.

I wrote the minister with dual responsibility for the PDD program and PPC Act portfolios. I shared our family's negative experience with the agency, identified misalignment with PDD values and acknowledged my allegation of emotional abuse.

I give the minister full credit for acknowledging shortcomings. The following is an excerpt from his response:

I commend your ongoing support and advocacy for your son, Matthew. He is fortunate to have a family that seeks creative options to support his independence in the community. It will take such advocacy, information, training and time for service providers and communities to better understand and embrace changes to what is a long-term approach to supporting people with developmental disabilities.

I'd met this minister in a few meetings, and he struck me as an ethical man. I sensed some heart and truth in his message, not empty words. Still, it wasn't a pat on the back that I sought. I wanted accountability and responsiveness from the system. Systems need to listen and respect—not dismiss—the voices of people they are paid to be serving. That approach works in theory, but isn't so commonplace in practice.

The ministerial letter and the PPC Act investigator's draft report coincidentally arrived at our home on the same day. Neil and I found it hard to reconcile how two personal documents representing the same ministry conveyed such different perspectives on our parental roles.

The minister's letter struck me as respectful, balanced and encouraging, while the administration's was the polar opposite. I believe that any reputable investigative process should consider differing perspectives, seek clarity and dig deeper to get the whole picture before passing judgement. But my experience differed. Like a street dog beaten and whimpering from repeated blows, I snapped back.

Once again, I wrote to the minister, voicing concerns about the overall investigative process. Knowing full well that senior PPC Act staff would be made aware of my ministerial correspondence, I chose words both carefully and unapologetically. The following is an excerpt from my second letter:

We had expected some good would come from this report. However, we are now hard pressed to find any value. The lesson we learned is how readily the voice of the dissenter is overruled and how service system logic trumps common sense. The report's recommendations reinforce agency rigidity and teach us a powerful lesson as to why families don't dare challenge the service system. Although we did provide a written response to the report, we could only bring ourselves to provide limited comments, as we are drained from the ordeal and have no more energy to invest.

It took another month before the final 28-page report was received by mail. I'd often seen the stock cover letters that accompanied lengthy PPC Act reports. This time the letter was addressed to me personally. It thanked me for reporting the allegation and was signed by the director, someone I worked closely with on committees. Salt rubbed into my raw wounds. The letter's closing comment stated, "It is the intention of the Act to better protect the health, safety and well-being of adults in care." Our son wanted to live life, not be *in care*—a distinction that the risk-aversive system missed.

Matt was deemed the perpetrator for challenging agency practices, getting mad and violating agency authority. It portrayed our son as nothing but a problem client. Specific examples of infractions cited included: changing the burned-out bulb, using de-icer and the unsolicited lawn mowing. Such a troublemaker!

I was painted as demanding, unrealistic and ignorant of any shortcomings of my son. I saw my biggest shortcoming as being unrealistic and ignorant about the agency's incapacity to take a leap forward, skin their knees and get up to stretch some more.

A rare explosion of profanity purged the vile venom that brewed in my gut throughout this ordeal. Feeling cleansed by the venting, I focused on moving forward.

Later I heard that other families complained about Craig's authoritative bullying and he left the agency. I wasn't interested in details. The less said about him the better.

We chose to rely solely on family, as deeply inflicted system fractures, cuts and bruises healed. Emotional recovery and the courage to trust again could not be rushed.

Chapter 29: Angelo's Journey

Leaving the family nest is a rite of passage into adulthood. But we were dealing with Mr. Enthusiasm. Matt embraced every opportunity to tell complete strangers his news. No details were spared.

"'Scuse me while I squeeze past. Cart's overflowing 'cause I'm moving out. Yup, gettin' my own apartment. Sure need to buy lots of stuff. Good thing my mum has her credit card. You do, right Mum?"

I smiled and shrugged my shoulders, grateful for a decent credit limit. My purse strings relaxed, knowing the spending surge wouldn't be reflected until the next billing cycle.

Matt's move to independent living marked a leap of faith. All family members eagerly awaited their next stage of life—increased independence. Kate, now 19 and a fresh high school graduate, travelled to Australia for a year with her future husband, Robby. Now a young woman she was bright, responsible, kind, and had a good head on her shoulders. At 23, Matt was eager for freedom—us too. The idea of being empty nesters was exhilarating.

The prospective apartment was both owned and operated by a traditional support agency. This small complex was the agency's first foray into supported independent living. I needed to be proactive, negotiate well and monitor vigilantly. When viewing the apartment, I initiated a probe.

"Matt's always had a cat and it's important he has one in his own place. Understandably he'd be fully responsible for its care. I want to confirm that it's allowed."

"Oh, don't think so, I'll take a peek." Daisy, the friendly project manager pulled the lease from her briefcase and scanned it quickly. "You know, surprisingly it doesn't specify."

I smiled and seized the moment. "Sounds to me like the lease allows for some discretion. That sure would go a long way in reassuring Matt."

Matt had wandered into the dingy kitchen. Faded green paint strokes representing three evergreen trees decorated the grungy feature wall. This was the sole remaining apartment in a neglected four-plex that the agency had recently bought. Volunteers from a local Rotary Club were updating the interior spaces. Renovating this apartment was their final chore.

Matt returned to the living room, clearly sitting on the fence. "I don't know, Mum. It's kinda…well, just not what I expected."

I glanced at Daisy. My raised eyebrows and tightly sealed lips sent an unspoken plea to sway Matt's decision. She replied with warm eyes.

"So Matt, this apartment will be fixed up, starting tomorrow and be ready within a week or so. Volunteers plan to clean and paint all weekend. It's yours if you want. But your mum indicated that not having a cat might be a deal breaker. Is that true?"

"Oh, yah. Need my cat."

"Well then, let's make a deal."

Daisy pulled out her pen and amended the lease, specifying that a cat was allowed. Matt's hesitancy dissolved when he signed the lease and was given his own copy for safekeeping.

With a stranglehold on his copy of the lease, Matt said "We'd better get shopping now, Mum."

Shopping trips to outfit his new apartment were plentiful and prolonged. Anything Matt identified as cool, handy or on sale always got close inspection. I was publicly cast in the role of tightwad mother. Master negotiation skills were applied by both parties. *Matt logic* assumed that graduating to apartment living should be accompanied by heaps of new stuff. Discussion of budget realities and the availability of decent furniture from home met resistance.

"But Mum, isn't that why you own a credit card?"

Weary with explanation, laden with "good deals" and burdened by a soaring credit card balance, we headed home. The most critical task of the day had intentionally been kept off the checklist. Scooter, his beloved favourite cat, would stay with our family. Conveying that news had to be done strategically, succinctly, and swiftly. The timing crystalized when Scooter rubbed against my leg during dinner.

"Our precious Scooter just reminded me to pass along a message. He won't be moving with you." Matt's head lifted from his plate. "Now hear me out. Scooter belongs to our whole family. You are starting a new life, so it would be nice to share that new life with a new pet, a kitten adopted from the animal shelter. They always have lots who need a loving home. Dad could take you Friday to have a look. Whatcha think?"

Within a nanosecond, Matt snatched up and soothingly consoled his feline soulmate. "Scooter, you know I'll always love you. But you belong here and I'm movin' out. Some little kitten needs me for a good home and lots of love—like I've always given you and your sister too."

He kissed Scooter, then spent all evening on the animal shelter website looking for the perfect kitten. Candidates abounded with interesting colours and markings. Our printer worked overtime, spewing individual pictures that completely covered his bed.

Matt was giddy with excitement on Friday morning. The ground rules were set and Neil was the enforcer, being much less malleable than me.

"Matt, remember you can take all the time you need to look at kittens in their cages. But you can't take any into the visiting room." We knew that holding a kitten would mark the point of no return. Having both Scooter and his shy littermate, Yuki, at home, nixed the prospect of introducing a kitten, even for a weekend sleepover.

"But Dad…."

"No buts. You can check out your favourites and then make your final choice after the weekend. That way you can take the kitten straight to your new apartment. Monday is your moving day, right?"

"It sure is. But if no kitten today, can we at least buy all the stuff we need? We'll need a travel case so it'll be safe in the car. And a litter box, kitty litter, food, bowl, collar...and at least one toy. See, I'm trying to save you guys money by not asking for lots of toys. We can always buy more later."

"Sounds like a good list. Shopping is your mum's territory though, so work that through with her." The weekend was a shopping frenzy.

Arriving long before the shelter opened on Monday morning, time dragged on. As staff unlocked the front door, Matt unlocked his seatbelt. With the cat carrier in hand, he proudly entered the facility to pick his treasure. Stopping dead in his tracks, Matt sensed something was amiss. He promptly found a staff person.

"It feels quiet here, like a library. On Friday my dad said all the meowing sounded like a jazz orchestra. My dad likes music. Did you move all the kittens out back?"

The answer from the young woman left us speechless. "I worked on Friday—and what a loud orchestra it was! We were bursting at the seams with kittens, so needed a plan. On Saturday morning, a friend at the radio station announced an impromptu 'adopt a kitten' day and gave it lots of airtime. The community's response was amazing. Almost all kittens were adopted." Her smile evaporated when she saw Matt's crestfallen face.

"Oh, but we do have two sweet little kittens left. Want to see them?"

Still dumbfounded by the news, Matt agreed. Then he turned his attention to me. "Told ya we should have picked a kitten on Friday," he muttered, shaking his head in disbelief.

The remaining kittens were identical male littermates—jet-black with zero markings. Our son's eyebrows jumped to his hairline, as if seeing double.

"Matt, think about it for a moment. Even though the kittens look the very same, they're unique, just like people," I reassured him. "Let's give them both a chance to show their personalities." Nodding to the staff, I asked if she could direct us to the visiting room.

All kittens are cute, and these were no exception. We had time alone with each furball to see how we bonded. The first kitten did little to interact. However, his brother was a different story. He purred incessantly, while sniffing and crawling all over Matt.

"Well, looks like he wanted to beat out his brother," Matt laughed. So began their love affair.

While we picked up our silky green-eyed beauty, Neil hastily delivered apartment furniture and boxes of essentials to unpack. I drove the roommates to their new home, enjoying the cooing concerto en route. Matt cradled his precious bundle, showing him every nook and cranny of the apartment. "Here's where we'll eat and you can sleep with me, like Scooter always did. And your litter box is right here." He nudged the kitten inside for a trial run.

"Look at him, Mum. He's such an angel. That's what I'll call him, Angel."

"You could, but it sounds more like a girl's name. Boy angels are often called Angelo instead."

"Huh, didn't know that. It does sound better. Welcome home. Angelo. I love you already."

Matt hated leaving Angelo alone when he went to his part-time job at Best Buy. Matt's last-minute work departures often meant a mad scramble to catch his bus on time. At 6:30 one weekday morning we got a frantic call.

"Sorry Mum—got an emergency! I stepped back when tying my work boot—right on Angelo's foot. He's crying lots. You need to come immediately so we can go to the vet. I'll have him ready in five minutes."

"Hold on—we're still in bed, the vet isn't open and it's probably a bad bruise."

"Mum! You're *not* listening! Can't you hear him crying? I'll hold him closer to the phone."

"No, that's not necessary; just let him rest. Better head out now or you'll be late for work. Dad can drop by later this morning and check Angelo."

"No. I've already called work and cancelled my shift. Left a message that I've got a family emergency. It's true—he is my family too. Oh Angelo, I'm so sorry. I didn't mean to hurt…" With his voice beginning to crack, he paused and drew some deep breaths.

"Matt. It'll be okay. Please, head off to work.…"

"Mum, I said no!" Those deep breaths had rekindled his passion for immediate action.

Admonishment followed on the heels of his frustrated sigh. "I'm *very* disappointed in you. If you guys don't know how to be responsible, I'll take Angelo to the vet, on the bus." The dial tone told me all I needed to know. Neil's eyes sought details.

"Sounds like Angelo's going on his first bus ride. Just another day in the Matt Lane." We sighed in two-part harmony.

The next call from the vet clinic was much calmer. Like we suspected, Angelo had a bad bruise. At Matt's request, the vet took an x-ray to confirm, then gave Angelo a shot for pain.

"Can you or Dad pick us up? Two bus rides in one day would traumatize Angelo. I had to convince the bus driver to even let him

284

on." Then in a hushed voice, "Hope I can borrow your credit card too. Get paid Tuesday and will try to pay you back then."

Matt's support agency and our family clashed over values, rhetoric, approaches and expectations. Entrenched group-home attitudes and practices lingered in the air and went unchallenged, except by us. Like a mismatched marriage, an adversarial relationship soon ruled the day. Matt and Angelo were asked to leave the agency-owned and operated four-plex after 21 months. The break-up was inevitable. As in a nasty divorce, both sides wiped their hands with a shared sense of good riddance.

My own government system espoused inclusion, yet didn't hold the agency to account. Feeling betrayed by an agency that created more stress than support, pursuing an alternate support agency felt too risky. I'd provide support as needed.

Serendipitously, a rare rental opportunity arose, in a small, attractive apartment complex around the corner from our home. The lawn sign stakes were still settling into the soil when we jumped on the opportunity. Matt and Angelo enjoyed a spacious one-bedroom apartment with a balcony, big windows and nice view. A far cry from their former residence which offered views of an adjacent apartment building wall or the back alley.

About 18 months after the move, a wonderful vacation opportunity arose. "I can't believe it! Uncle Mike actually bought me an airline ticket to visit everyone in the Maritimes. Flying so far and all by myself—like, wow!"

"You're lucky to have such a generous uncle. You'll have 10 days to visit my brothers, your grandma and aunties. Dad and I'll take that time for our own vacation. Don't worry, Kate and Robby said they can look after Angelo."

Our daughter Kate and her husband Robby had recently moved back to Edmonton and lived close by. Being avid pet lovers, they agreed to visit Angelo daily for feeding, snuggling and litter box changes. What sounded like a simple and effective plan to us was anything but for Angelo. After a few visits, Robby came home one evening and shared an unsettling experience.

"As crazy as this sounds, when I filled Angelo's cat dish, he hissed and charged, swatting at me." Somewhat embarrassed, Robby added, "It felt like Angelo had suddenly turned feral. I actually used the bristles of the nearby broom to keep him at bay when shutting the door."

"You've got to be kidding me," Kate chortled. "Angelo is a gentle sweetheart. Sure it wasn't your imagination?" Robby's look confirmed that he wasn't joking.

The next day Kate visited sweetheart Angelo and her experience was strikingly similar to Robby's. Angelo's foul mood remained, as did the broom by the door. His daily basic needs were met until we returned from our holidays. Poor Angelo was in solitary confinement.

What hadn't crossed my mind when planning our trip was that Angelo had been abandoned as a kitten. Although Matt left his beloved cat only once before, it was for two days to visit a college friend in Calgary. During that time I spent quality time with Angelo, who knew me extremely well. The cat clearly missed Matt then, but managed fine. Angelo didn't have the same comfort level with Kate and Robby.

This extended vacation had emotionally traumatized Angelo, triggering a slow downward spiral. He wasn't as content, became less interested in snuggling and developed a tendency to swat visitors. This made people uneasy, including me.

"Here Mum, say hello to Angelo," Matt said, innocently thrusting an uncooperative Angelo into my face.

"No Matt—he's obviously not comfortable, so neither am I."

"But he's your grandcat, so it should be fine."

"I know, but still, if he doesn't want to be picked up.…"

"This is getting really frustrating," Matt grumbled. "I don't know why Angelo doesn't like people like he used to. I've started giving him timeouts when he swats at anybody. He doesn't feel like the same cat anymore."

Matt started his own downward spiral, leaving Angelo alone for longer periods during the day. "He's okay on his own, Mum. I always make sure he has food and water. That's all he needs."

"Oh Matt. He needs your love and attention." My lips moved, but fell on deaf ears. Like squabbling best friends, Matt and Angelo's happiness waned and indifference to each other mounted.

After two years or more, the apron strings of dependence that I'd worked so hard to snip through independent living had become tightly re-knotted. Matt was definitely living a slovenly bachelor's life, with little attention to household management. Dirty dishes were piled on every kitchen surface, clean and dirty clothes intermingled on his bedroom floor and papers galore carpeted his living room. He'd slipped far from his initial enthusiasm to keep his place looking and feeling good. Each knot of dependence was incrementally tightened with mutual resentment.

"Matt, how can you even find the table to eat on? Maybe not an issue since there's not a clean dish in sight. And nothing but empty hangers in your closet. Tons of clothes on your floor though. You need to do better...a lot better!"

"It's not that bad. Did two loads of laundry then took a nap. Must've kicked them off the bed, mixing them up with dirty clothes. We could sniff them and then hang up the clean ones. Need more loonies to wash sheets too. Got some?"

"No! This is your responsibility Matt, not mine. Look, Angelo's lying on work pants. Clean or not, now they're covered in pet hair. And your work shift is in two hours. Shake them out and grab a lint brush...if you can find one."

Matt intended to keep commitments, but lacked focus. Plans rarely materialized unless the event was both important *and* exciting enough to command his undivided attention. Being the deepest sleeper I know, risks of Matt missing important appointments ran high. I tried to keep track, reminding him when appointments were imminent. After several unsuccessful reminder calls it was not uncommon for me to ring his bell, then resort to using my key. Dead to the world, I'd shake his shoulder, leg and then whole body, while calling him loudly. The bed vibrated with his snoring. Eventually he'd wake and I'd end up driving him blurry eyed to his appointment. Exhaustion and impatience consumed me. Matt wasn't physically living at home, but he gobbled my time and energy. I needed to take another leap of faith and snip those badly knotted apron strings.

After considerable soul searching, I hesitantly re-engaged agency support, with an organization that walked the talk of citizenship and inclusion. Despite their tremendous dedication and creative efforts to re-engage Matt in community life, he remained isolated and overly reliant on me. So the agency suggested a different approach.

The proposal was to match Matt with Fletcher, a well-respected staff person. Together they'd find a decent two-bedroom apartment and live as roommates, sharing rent. The goal was to reduce Matt's growing social isolation. Intellectually I understood the potential benefits. Positive, accepting and a cool guy, Fletcher had the endorsement of our whole family.

Matt liked Fletcher and contemplated the idea. "I'm okay with it so long as we pick the place together and Angelo gets to come too." So it was agreed.

My gut was still uneasy, something I felt compelled to share. "Even with such a dream roommate, it's a huge gamble to give up Matt's affordable, convenient and pet-friendly apartment. What if the arrangement doesn't work out? We'd be hard pressed to match his current rental." While nobody had a backup plan, everyone agreed that quality of life was significantly declining for Matt and Angelo.

We held our breath and hesitantly gave notice. The guys found a suitable place and signed a one-year lease. The feasibility of continuing the arrangement would be reviewed before the year ended. I recalled taking such a gamble in my young adulthood— with someone I hadn't even met.

After fulfilling his one-year roommate agreement, Fletcher was exhausted by the breadth and depth of Matt's ever undulating support challenges. Needing time to rejuvenate and reclaim his personal autonomy, Fletcher chose not to renew the living arrangement with Matt. Through nobody's fault, the roommate gamble failed.

Matt couldn't afford to keep the apartment on his own, nor could the agency find a reasonably priced decent one-bedroom that was pet-friendly. Matt adamantly refused to consider a bachelor apartment, which was what he could afford.

"No, no, no Mum! It's just not fair! If I have to move I need a one-bedroom like before. I will *not* consider anything less." It was like he was wearing headphones that blocked out a deafening alarm bell. The dire situation eluded him while the relentless alarm intensified in our heads.

On the last day of the lease, Matt walked out the door, abandoning Angelo and his belongings for the agency to address. As inconceivable as it was, I stood united with the agency and my family. Rescuing Matt would only perpetuate the cycle of dependence. The agency was willing to help him explore housing options when he was ready. Matt's wall of rage was impenetrable. He called everyone's bluff, but nobody blinked.

Once again Angelo was abandoned and destined for darkness, or so I thought. Rather than returning Angelo to the animal shelter where his demise would most likely be imminent, this agency went the extra mile. Nicola, the agency's executive director, found someone to foster Angelo in a loving home.

Matt did visit Angelo a few times. "You'd be amazed, Mum. He lives in a house with other cats and they all get along. Other cats— and there's no swatting! Angelo even gets to go outside for the first time in his life and he likes the independence. He sat on my lap for a few minutes but then wanted to go be with his new buddies. That's okay. I understood."

Both Matt and his cat were survivors of troubling times. It gave me comfort to know that in Angelo's latter years, this gentle feline once again enjoyed security, companionship and love. Shortly after regaining stability in his life, Matt hesitantly asked a surprising question.

"Now that I have an apartment again, think I should ask to have Angelo back?" I sensed reluctance, mixed with guilt.

"Well, knowing about Angelo's life now, what do you think?" I prayed for a glimpse of insight.

"Ya know Mum, I think Angelo's got it good where he lives now. Living in an apartment with me, he couldn't go outside."

"That's true. So how do you think being housebound would make him feel?"

"I think he'd miss the freedom he has now—bet it would make him sad." Matt stared into space for a moment, processing his thoughts. "Can't do that to him. Guess I'll be happy knowing that he's happy. Good ol' Angelo...."

Chapter 30: Money, Money, Money

Matt likes simple solutions. No cash? No problem. That's where cheques, payday loan companies, credit cards and pawnshops come in handy. With outstretched tentacles they offer enticing breadcrumbs of immediate gratification. Matt's realities of executive functioning challenges, living in the moment and impulsivity provide a recipe for disaster. His chance of not being lured into debt is slim at best. The concept of repayment poses no perceivable threat, seemingly far away. Filed under "Later."

Matthew opened his first initial "Fat Cat" savings account at our local credit union when he was 10. He loved stepping up to the teller, all of whom he knew by name. Our entrepreneurial lad carefully counted bills and pulled loose change from his pocket. With fingers strangling the pen and tongue poking from the corner of his mouth, he focused intently on legibly signing the back of customer cheques.

Deposits represented the hard-earned income from his fledgling lawn and snow shovelling business. Withdrawals, made as separate transactions immediately after deposits, represented the reward for hard work.

One afternoon, at age 12, Matthew arrived home with his deposit slip and customary Slurpee, plus a colourful notice. Sitting at the kitchen table he read the details of a contest for young account holders. Entrants needed to write a mini essay about their responsible saving. The prize was an enticing $250 bursary. Matthew's submission still rings true over two decades later.

I have been getting into a habit of taking money out of my account to spend it on junk food and trying to get out of this habit. I think I sould save up my money that I earn with my Buissness. There are things that I want to buy that I don't have the money for and whant to get it. I have not secseeded by meetin the head start criteria goal. From now on before I take money out of my account that I sould think about what I am spending it on.

291

Matthew typed up this entry on his business letterhead, which acknowledged that he didn't meet the contest criteria. Did he think that nobody else would be applying? His logic eluded me, but made sense to him.

After turning 16, Matt talked with the bank about getting his own cheques. His request was granted. He was thrilled, while I was not. For a few days I grappled with bursting his bubble. I resented knowing that I'd likely need to wrestle the cheque book from his control. Then I noticed two were missing.

"Matt, I know you're excited about having a chequebook, but it's not so easy to keep under control."

"I'm sure I can do it. Only wrote two so far. I mailed a cheque today to the Red Cross 'cause I saw on TV that some people are starving. You know I'll always help. I borrowed an envelope and stamp from your writing desk."

"Helping others is always good, but how much money is in your bank and how much was the cheque you wrote?"

"Well this one was for $20 and I wrote one yesterday at Safeway for pop and treats. I think that was about $10."

"And how much money do you have in your bank from snow shovelling?"

"I deposited $30 on Monday, then took out $5 for lunch at McDonald's."

"Matt, that leaves about $25 in your account. The cheques for the Red Cross and Safeway add up to more than that. The bank will bounce one and then you'll be charged money."

"No, no, no Mum. You don't understand. The biggest cheque I wrote was $20. I just can't write a cheque for more than $25. So I'll still have $5 left in the bank. Don't think the 7-Eleven would let me write a cheque for a Slurpee, so not even gonna try."

My headache became full-blown and Matt offered to get me an Aspirin. The chequebook disappeared shortly thereafter, but a cheque bounced in the interim.

When finishing high school, Matt was delighted to receive a pre-approved low-limit credit card in the mail. This financial gift from corporate scalpers reinforced Matt's rights, as someone who recently reached adulthood. Ramifications unfolded rapidly.

I needed to rectify this immediately. In a brief moment of clarity Matt agreed to me calling the company. I waited on hold for almost a half hour. Meanwhile Matt wandered away. A woman with a heavy Texan drawl eventually greeted me. She was distant in both location and empathy.

"But you don't understand. My son did not request this credit card. Besides having an intellectual disability, he lacks impulse control and the financial means to pay it off. Please cancel it now. My son's at home. I'll quickly nab him so he can tell you directly."

"I'm sorry ma'am but I have other calls to answer. Our policy is to congratulate all high school grads by giving them the opportunity to build good credit. You'll notice the card's lower credit limit to encourage responsible spending."

The flash of anger in my eyes shot into my voice. "Ah yes, I noticed the extremely high interest too. Perhaps your company frames that as a deterrent to maxing out the credit card?"

"Actually, it can be just that. Well ma'am if he doesn't want the card he can cut it up. I can't help anymore than I have. Y'all have a good day now."

Hanging up in disgust, I overheard Matt say goodbye and close the front door.

"Hungry, Mum? Got us pizza for lunch. Signed for it with my new credit card."

"Oh Matt! We talked about the importance of cancelling that card before you used it."

"You were on the phone too long, and I was hungry. Was impressed with the super fast delivery time, so naturally I included a good tip."

"On the other hand, I'm far from impressed with your actions."

"Jeez, Mum—stop worrying so much! I'm sure I can handle it. Card's even got my name on it." He proudly slipped the card into his wallet, tucking it safely away from my maternal grip. Credit felt like income—manna from heaven.

Pizza and other take-out delivery drivers rang our bell for lunch and dinner daily, until the card was maxed out—within a week. Like nudging a toboggan precariously perched on a mountaintop, the piles of take-out boxes signalled the beginning of his perilous and reckless descent into financial disaster.

Life in the Matt Lane is not for the faint of heart. It has been daunting, educational and insightful for those who advocate and are committed to stand by his side. Like living in Hurricane Alley, all can be deadly calm, then suddenly all hell breaks loose. The pressure of the storm can crack our family's protective shell, splitting it wide open.

As Mum, I tried various strategies to influence Matt financially, without being overbearing. He increasingly balked at any guidance, spending all income on day one and then being broke. When calmness returned, he often agreed on a weekly allotment that would ensure funding throughout the month. Spouting responsibility strategies and enacting them never aligned.

Matt routinely got stuck, perseverating on his rights and fanning the emotional flame. With closed ears and a red face, he'd yell. "It's my money, so *nobody* can tell me how to spend it. I want every penny of it—now! I'm prepared to call the police on you."

We didn't want control over Matt's money but realistic options for others to do so were lacking. We were fortunate when a colleague's sister, an empathetic banking advisor, took Matt under her wing. Matt's weekly appointments with his personal advisor gave him a sense of pride and importance. She was consistently realistic, clear and forthright with our son about responsible financial management. He liked her, but tired of the clear messages, so transferred to another bank, then another and another.

Matt's understanding of banking has improved with age. However, like Swiss cheese, his brain has deep logic holes, landing him in overdraft situations that he never anticipates or comprehends. With limited funds for the basics of life, society's focus on consumerism drew our son into the world of greedy moneylenders, pawnshops and victimization by supposed friends. He began to know employee names at pawnshops and payday loan companies. Impulsivity and poor choices were rationalized in the moment. Without grasping the consequences of his actions, bizarre events unfolded.

One such example stemmed from his roommate Fletcher refusing to loan Matt money to buy a two-litre Coke. Our son fixated on needing the Coke and employed *Matt logic*. He'd show Fletcher. Unplugging his large flat-screen TV, Matt waited at the bus stop, awkwardly manoeuvred it on and off the bus, then walked a block to the pawnshop. After initially telling me the TV was being repaired, he finally came clean.

"You've got to be kidding me! Giving up your much-loved TV for a pop? You know the drill—paying ridiculously high interest rates and losing valuable belongings when pawn fees skyrocket. Over and over, again, and again…and again." I started to sob.

"Please, don't cry Mum, please. I know it was stupid. Promise to get it back soon." But he didn't.

Financial disasters and anxiety piled high like stinking garbage. In a society that entices with "you deserve" and "great deals," moneylenders and pawnshop loans masquerade as solutions, not problems. And signing one's name on a contract feels good—until the hounds are called in to collect. Creditors ramped up pressure, threatening legal action. That daily pressure skyrocketed anxiety. Inconceivably we were advised that there was only one card left to play. Bankruptcy was on the table.

Shortly after all was settled and pressure relieved, Matt and I were walking past a Money Mart. He slowed and nonchalantly inquired, "Mum do you think I should go in and ask about a payday loan?"

"Omigod—no! Why would you even consider that?"

"I don't know...well, maybe just in case?" The lesson from his painful and prolonged angst already eluded his grasp.

Bone weary, I watched my grown lamb stumble, fall, get up and repeat. Like that song by Canadian rock band Rush, I felt like Matt was "working them angels overtime." Financial woes continued, despite Matt having a part-time job.

Promise showed on the horizon while sitting on a cross-ministerial committee charged with creating an informal trustee program for people who had significant challenges managing their government-funded disability allowances. Until then, Alberta's Office of the Public Trustee (OPT) had only served people with significant financial assets. That changed with the adoption of an informal trustee program. The service helped people who struggled with financial management by having their disability allowance distributed through the OPT. Matt consented to this, but became annoyed with how their effective budgeting strategies limited his spending. Upon learning that he could withdraw consent for the informal trusteeship arrangement by simply signing a form, he wasted no time. His withdrawal catapulted us into dark, familiar territory.

Matt was swirling in a deep financial quagmire when I heard exciting news related to the Registered Disability Savings Funds. Our annual financial contributions were accumulating in a time capsule. Those funds, held on Matt's behalf could be considered financial assets under OPT policy if the accumulated amount met the eligibility threshold. And it did! Elated, I anticipated a straightforward process. But theory and reality spoke different languages.

For two full years I bared my soul and pleaded to get a public trustee appointed. The system required a formal "capacity assessment" completed by a designated professional, such as his physician or a psychologist. Knowing Matt since infancy, our family's general practitioner understood and appreciated my concerns. However, he struggled with the ethics of completing the assessment report against our adult son's wishes. In letters to both the OPT and family doctor I wrote: "Matt is on a very slippery slope. I'm terrified that he'll be destitute and homeless if this excruciatingly stalled process takes much longer."

Both professionals were empathetic yet stymied by personal ethics, policy and legal processes. An independent adult in the eyes of the courts, Matt refused to see a psychologist for assessment, convinced he could manage his funds. I consulted with psychologists to no avail. "Just let me know if he changes his mind" offered no consolation.

Preparing a trusteeship application prior to Matt's clock striking adulthood could have saved us great anguish, while leaving Matt bitter over being controlled. We reluctantly gave Matt ample opportunities to exercise basic financial independence. Yet, eventually we all need to pay the piper and the debt compounds with time.

Matt's emotional state grew fragile as his roommate arrangement with Fletcher drew to a close. Anxiety, tension and indignation soared. Refusing all guidance and logic, Matt plunged into a deep, dark well of homelessness. We prayed that bone-numbing water would shock him back towards sunshine—but when? Taking the lead and setting the direction rested with Matt. Guidance can't be forced, just offered—a harsh reality for all adults.

After a lengthy, unwarranted stint in shelters, Matt gradually renewed contact with Nicola's support agency and reluctantly agreed to a capacity assessment. That was the key to achieving the long-awaited security of legal trusteeship.

Challenges have been greatly reduced since having legal trusteeship in place. Matt can still step into financial quagmires but the severity of risks has been greatly diminished. Having our family removed from the middle of financial battles has lifted a great burden from our shoulders. Like a broken record we repeated the same message until it was finally received, needing only occasional reinforcement.

"Matt, you're talking to the wrong person. Your family's here to love and support you, not to be involved with your finances. Work it through with the trustee."

"Then I'll go to their office and cancel it, just like before."

"Not an option. Remember, this time it was a judge who made the decision, in court. Overturning it would require a long legal process and nobody other than you would support it. Certainly not your family."

He threw up his hands. "So frustrating! Wish I'd never agreed to that stupid assessment!"

"Oh, Matt. Every human being has areas in life where they struggle—your dad and me too. Trouble handling money is a whopper for you."

"You're not listening! I'm *sure* I can do it this time." He exhaled a long sigh then added, "I was successful before."

"Okay, I'll try to listen better. When did you manage your money well?"

"When I was living in homeless shelters." Frantically, I searched for words.

"Matt, how can you say that? In shelters you didn't have to pay rent or buy food. Even then, you still spent your monthly disability cheque within a single day."

298

"Doesn't matter—only bought good-quality stuff."

It was useless to delve deeper.

Having a legal trustee appointed ensures basics are covered, provides parameters and mitigates risks. Vigilance and oversight are as good as it gets.

Chapter 31: Give Me Shelter

Tattered, torn and terrified summed it up. Matt was adrift, shivering in line at the homeless shelter, seeking a hot meal and a mat to sleep on. There was no need for him to be homeless. If only he'd listened to reason when his roommate arrangement with Fletcher ended. Finding an affordable one-bedroom apartment was out of his reach. Indignation at the prospect of a bachelor apartment, coupled with certainty that Mum would bail him out, didn't serve him well. Out of options, the homeless shelter awaited.

I've always empathized with people who are homeless and struggling on the streets. Each one was once someone's beautiful little baby. Somewhere along the way life's traumas and challenges took a heavy toll. Discarded, shunned and desperate on so many levels. This societal group of invisible souls now had a new member, our vulnerable son. Our family joined the ranks of distressed families who live with the anguish of loved ones who slipped from their loving embrace, into the depths of homelessness. Unacknowledged sleepless nights for all.

Seeing me staring blankly out the window on this cold rainy day, Kate thrust her young babe into my arms. "Here, Mum. Hug Devyn. Long as you want—anytime." Walking away she cheekily added, "Hey, she could even sleep in your bedroom tonight. Whatcha think?" I smiled weakly in response.

"Just kiddin'—hand her back whenever you want." A freshly minted mother, Kate had a new appreciation of my angst over her brother's precarious situation.

Absorbing my precious granddaughter's unconditional love warmed the vast aching hole in my heart. While I was taking comfort in cradling Kate's firstborn, mine was aimlessly wandering the streets. How did we arrive here? A simple question, without a simple answer.

Family realities are like intricate tapestries. Carefully crafted details convey a distinct image on the surface. However, the flipside reveals a tangled, crisscrossed mess of threads and knots. That mess reflects the real story—a creation formed through blood, sweat and tears. Tapestry threads are finely woven and hard to untangle. The rear view never reconciles with the tidy public image. Even on the surface, our family tapestry was stark, grim and screaming to be addressed. Naïve well-wishers thought Matt's homelessness could be easily dealt with. Just add an extra tapestry stitch and find him shelter. Superficially so simple. Deep dives into *why* revealed caverns of complexity.

"What—Matt's wandering the streets? As parents, how can you let him be out there? Where will he go? You're going to get him, right?"

"Actually no, we're not. Hard as that is to imagine—well—living it is so much worse...." My voice drifted away with each word, detaching emotionally, while physically present.

Most didn't have good poker faces. At best, people were perplexed and disappointed that we weren't rushing to the rescue. Nobody offered any viable solutions. Still they were convinced that our family had to *do something*.

They pressed relentlessly. "So what about the risks? With desperate people aplenty he's *so* easy to prey upon. You're okay with that?"

Silently I bellowed: "Leave me alone!" There was enough self-flagellation going on. In a flatline manner, I responded, "This is the hardest thing we've done in our lives." Vacant eyes begged them to walk away.

Our family drifted in a sea of uncertainty. We were united in knowing that playing the saviour role wouldn't yield insights or emotional stability for Matt. Turning our backs and waiting for him to take some semblance of ownership for his situation was the only way. The tremendous risks of that stance frightened us all. Neil was stoic on the surface while I was visibly distraught. Underneath it all we were entwined in worry. We would only survive this gale by linking arms on a small but sturdy life raft.

Nicola, the committed executive director of the agency that had supported Matt, remained peripherally involved, even though he'd walked away from their offers of help. Unbeknownst to Matt, when waiting in the shelter line-up, she watched from her car discreetly parked down the street.

"Susan, I know this is hard," Nicola said, "but you need to stay strong. Once Matt agrees, we can help him manage his money and find a place within his budget. Until then, our hands are tied."

Words poured from my heart. "I worried about challenges when the roommate arrangement ended, but this nightmare was inconceivable—until now."

With facts already stated, Nicola offered kindness. "If it'll help you sleep at night, let me assure you that I touch base with shelter staff routinely. They're good about keeping a watchful eye over him. And I wait until I see him get safely inside before heading home for dinner."

I did sleep easier knowing that there were silent guardians watching out for him. Still, I wrestled with how great promise had evaporated like mist on the mountains of hope. Days stretched into weeks, then months.

During lunch with Patti, a kind-hearted colleague, she said, "It must feel like salt being rubbed in open wounds. Your job assessing the quality of life for adults with developmental disabilities takes you into their homes. All the while you have to worry about Matt's homelessness."

"Ironic, but far from funny. After work, I see people waiting for buses to go home. Matt rides buses to nowhere all day, passing time until the shelter opens." My voice began to quake, "It's so hard...."

Patti squeezed my hand and took a few bites before continuing. "It's been a few months now…do you think he's finally hit rock bottom?"

"Thought I knew what rock bottom was, until he started this free fall into the dark realm of homelessness. I've learned the depth of my ignorance about geology. What I called rock bottom really wasn't—it was only multiple layers of silt, sand and clay. There are so many sinkholes that go deeper. I pray that he reaches bedrock soon. That solid base is what Matt needs to propel him towards stability. Think I've aged years in a matter of months."

"If you ever need a shoulder to lean on or someone to hold your hand as you scream, I'm here. There are lots of other people in your corner too."

My brimming eyes thanked her. "Speaking of people in my corner, let me tell you something—timing couldn't be worse though. Ages ago, I promised Darcy Elks to help facilitate this weekend's discussions with parents completing Social Role Valorization training." With my elbows on the table, outstretched digits of both hands cradled my head.

Patti dropped her fork. "Omigod! You're still going to do it? That would be so courageous."

"I respect Darcy too much to back out, so I called her. She thinks our plight is important to share and will be enlightening for people. My reward will be drinking from her elixir of empathy, understanding and commitment. Wish me luck."

I was one of two parents co-facilitating group discussions under Darcy's direction. Both of us were struggling significantly with young adult sons who had made ghastly choices of late. Not uncommon for young adults seeking independence and winding their way into the fullness of adulthood. Adulthood's fusion of independence and responsibility eluded our sons at that time. We took comfort from each other.

Our sons needed to find their sea legs and actively swim, rather than be transported across the water, cocooned as children in men's bodies. Both families emitted feint bursts of illumination, like lighthouses calling in darkness, timeworn beacons of inclusion. Standing on solid rock we waited for our sons to navigate their way through thick fog.

The weekend program started with every participant giving an overview of current challenges and triumphs. The pattern emerged quickly. Parents tried matching the first enthusiastically delivered experience, which was justly a cause of pride and celebration. In turn, each person shared a positive, uplifting incident, no matter how small. Any reference to challenges or setbacks were glossed over or avoided. As the last workshop participant wrapped up everyone was feeling stoked.

My turn was next. With my right hand over my heart, I looked at Darcy, bit my lip and hung my head. A collective air of confusion filled the room. I could do this—but needed to gather the gumption to do so.

Darcy's voice caressed me like angel wings. "Whenever you're ready, Susan." Wrapped in her empathy and encouragement, it was time.

"Okay, I um…." I took a deep breath and lifted my head. "Everyone's shared good stories, as I have in the past. But today…my heart is broken. My son's capabilities and accomplishments are buried under an avalanche of harsh reality." Through tears I managed to form and speak more words. "He is particularly at risk, and…and homeless."

I only heard chairs scrape on the tile floor—blinded by tears. Within moments I was enveloped by hugs, soothing words and non-judgemental caring. As my vision cleared, I noticed a man hanging back. He looked reluctant, yet eager to approach, shuffling his feet, awaiting an opportunity to engage me. When he did step forward, his face immediately crumbled.

Struggling to remain coherent, he gushed despair. "You're…you're living my worst nightmare…." Then he burst into deep cathartic sobs. The tables instantaneously turned. It was my turn to stand up and be the consoler. Not the session icebreaker that anyone had expected.

The dreaded weekend workshop became a welcome nourishing refuge. A good reminder that even when feeling alone, we're never alone. The opportunity for full disclosure in this safe environment massaged the paralysis from muscles seized by worry.

While staying at the shelter, Matt had full control over his monthly disability cheque. It took over two years to get a public trustee appointed by the courts. Until that proclamation he spent every disability cheque the day he received it. He purchased good-quality belongings to make his untenable situation more comfortable. Such items rarely lasted long in a place where desperation and exploitation are rampant. Matt didn't see that flaunting prized items made him a target for theft, or worse.

Initially our family curtailed all direct communication, emotionally safeguarding our stance. Gradually we reintroduced limited phone contact, to reinforce family connections before Matt drifted too far. We shared our eagerness to reward *any* initiative on his part. After a few months we opened our home and hearts to Sunday dinners with Matt.

One wintery Sunday shortly after getting his cheque, Matt arrived for dinner. He was proudly sporting a good-quality winter jacket and nice toque.

Never at a loss for words Kate quipped, "Matt, you're the best dressed homeless person I've ever seen."

"Okay…? So does that mean you like it? Think I chose a good colour. It'll help me stay warm when lined up in the freezing cold. Wish they'd let us in earlier."

"It is nice and should keep you warm too. Probably took all your money though. You'll need to keep a close eye on it so it doesn't get stolen."

"Don't worry. I'm keeping it right by me when I sleep."

"Good luck with that. Wasn't last month's expensive pillow stolen even though you slept on it?"

"Well yah. Someone stole it when I went to the bathroom. Only left it for a minute…."

I interjected, "Okay you two. Table needs setting—dinner's almost ready."

Working behind the scenes, Nicola leveraged her community connections and Matt was shortlisted for placement in YMCA housing. With a public trustee finally appointed, payment of his monthly rent would be assured. Matt slowly inched up the list.

One day an excited Matt called, with words tumbling over each other. "Good, good news! I've got a room at the YMCA and can move in this week."

"Oh Matt, that gives me shivers of joy! Dad and Kate will be so…"

His runaway train cut me off. "I'll have a private room and share the kitchen with other people on my floor. Everyone just needs to wash their dishes right away and keep the kitchen clean."

"Now you won't need to rush back after Sunday dinner. Your room and bed will always be waiting for you."

"Oh boy, I can hardly wait to sleep on a real bed again. Finally I'll get decent sleep. Some of those guys at the shelter snore even louder than me."

"And my dear, we all know you snore like a freight train." I sensed lightness on both ends of the phone.

"And no more waiting outside in the cold! Gonna call Martin next. Wait 'til Cuz hears this! Gotta go."

After hanging up, I breathed a deep sigh of relief and let the news absorb into my soul. I promptly called Neil and Kate, before sharing with colleagues, stopping at every office door.

Getting settled in the YMCA and having a public trustee to manage income marked the ascent from bedrock. Matt began to feel more settled. When dropping him back at the facility after dinner, it was not uncommon to see unsavoury characters and shady goings on outside their doors. This was definitely a step up, but far from a desirable arrangement.

One Sunday Matt asked to speak individually and in private with Neil, Kate, Robby and me before dinner. It seemed to be his way of acknowledging the challenges of his troublesome times. He shared different things depending on who he was talking to. With his dad he shared distressing and scary things he'd witnessed at the shelter. I'm glad he spared me such details.

He talked with me about being aware of how other people were struggling too. He mentioned getting to know a woman staying across the hall, with her two teenagers. It was news to me that besides housing men, the YMCA sheltered families too.

Matt shared that he spent $10 monthly on a Netflix account. Because he felt bad for this woman and her bored teens, he shared his account code with them. Always on high alert, I grilled him on how this arrangement came about. I wanted to ensure it wasn't foreshadowing being taken advantage of in some way.

"Oh Mum. Really, they're nice and in a tough spot. I'm happy to help." I let it slide.

After several months the public trustee saved enough funds for a damage deposit. Elated, Matt moved into an apartment again. Bordering on a sketchy part of town, it was a coveted one-bedroom and close to bus routes.

One day shortly after his move, Matt and I met downtown. Before heading home on our respective buses, he suggested we wait at the bus stop next to the Y.

As we approached the bus stop, we heard someone yell: "Hey, Matt!"

"What the heck!" Looking around he asked, "Who was that and were they calling me?"

"Not sure, Matt. I heard it too but don't see anyone. Maybe someone recognized you from a window in the Y. Or maybe it was meant for another Matt."

A few minutes later while still awaiting our buses, a woman ran across the street, headed in our direction. As she got closer, she beamed and waved. There was a certain swagger about her.

"Well, well. Matt, it is you. When you didn't answer I thought maybe I was mistaken." I had no idea who this person was.

"Mum, this is Iris. I met her at the Y when we both lived there. Iris, this is my mum, Susan."

Lived there? Maybe he misspoke. If he'd told me she was staff that would fit, but another resident? This woman was well dressed, confident and outgoing.

Iris said, "Oh yah, glad those days are behind us, hey Matt?" He nodded. "Your son was a gift to me and my kids when we were having a turbulent time."

308

"Matt mentioned a family living across the hall from him. That was you?"

"Sure was. My kids still talk about Matt sharing his Netflix code. In a way he was like our guardian angel. Being kind and watching out for my kids helped lighten my load."

Matt joined in. "When I saw how bored the kids were, it felt right to share."

"But we got off to a pretty rough start, right Matt?" She grinned and nudged him, rocking his body with her sturdy shoulder.

"I guess we kinda did," he fessed up, while colour crept up his face.

"You see," Iris said, "Matt *farted* when we were cooking in the kitchen and I thought that was pretty rude." She was forthright and assumed full ownership of her no-holds-barred approach. It made me grin. "Matt apologized later and it was very sincere. So we wiped the slate clean and started afresh."

Ah, yes, I mused. That damn elastin gene affects all muscles, large and small.

"Oh, Iris, I shouldn't be surprised that you outed me to my mum. We sure did get along." Playfully wagging his finger, he added, "And you have to agree we had no more kitchen incidents."

"Thank heavens. Hope you told your mum about being my saviour after that guy assaulted me."

"God no!" he reacted, zapped at the very suggestion.

"Well then, I will. Your son was the sole gentleman in a group of well over a hundred men. One asshole in particular kept eyeing my teenage daughter and making lewd comments. I called him on it, which pissed him off. Later he caught me alone in the elevator and beat me up."

"Despicable bastard!" I retorted. The thought of it made my blood boil.

"I want you to know that it was this young man right here who came to my assistance. He had staff call 911, got me a blanket and held my hand until the paramedics came. You've raised an extremely kind, gentle soul and should be proud of how he helps others."

"Matt's always been compassionate and jumps in whenever someone needs help. I must admit, your recognition warms my heart. Is it okay to give you a hug?"

"Absolutely. Don't get enough of them." The hug felt mutually reciprocated and welcomed.

"Well Matt, I see my bus up the street. Gotta run. Nice seeing you both!" Then Iris was gone. The memory of meeting her remains to this day.

Near the end of Matt's one-year lease he talked about renewal. Neil and I yearned for something different. If only we could pull it off. Like most families, we always craved the security of a permanent home for our vulnerable loved one. Reality taunted endlessly, reminding us that such security was financially beyond our means. However, a recent dip in the real estate market provided a glimmer of hope. The slump included a glut of basic apartments in older buildings that had been converted into condominiums.

Maybe the stars were aligning. If we could scrape together a down payment and have Matt's rent cover most of the mortgage payment.... The very idea made my heart flutter. I had to stall Matt's eagerness to renew, without unduly raising his hopes, or ours.

"Matt, there are still a couple of months on your lease so don't rush into renewing. Your dad and I are hoping to find something better that's still affordable."

"Well it would be nice to live someplace where I don't hear police sirens all night. If you go on the internet, you'll see the crime report for this area. I check it every week and it's not pretty. Your area's so much quieter."

"I know. Your dad and I are actively searching for something better. I promise we'll get things figured out before your renewal deadline." He agreed to hang tight, after many assurances that he wouldn't end up homeless again.

Much to our delight, our research and creative budgeting paid off. We found a well-constructed older building at a cost that we could manage. This midsize complex was in a desirable and familiar area, not far from our home. The condo was bright, spacious, on a quiet street, and had multiple bus options a few steps away.

I broached the subject with Matt by phone. "Here's how it would work. Dad and I would own the condo. We'd charge an affordable rent and you'd be expected to respect the condo as your very own home. We'd be going out on a limb for you, so before we consider putting in an offer you'd need to see and like the place."

"Hmm, you've sure kept this a good secret. Definitely like the idea. Hang on a minute, Mum. I know the location, but give me the *exact* address." I could hear him repeating the street numbers, while typing. "Yah, just like I thought. The crime rate statistics are really low there—as good as yours. How soon can I see it?"

Our whole family did the walk-through with our real estate friend, Colleen. The potential was evident so we decided to make an offer. Colleen and I conferred in the kitchen, while Matt was busy opening cupboard doors and turning on the faucet.

Colleen asked, "Now, do you want to have a home inspection first? Since it's a relatively small and vacant space it would be easy to just check things yourself. And of course, we'll get detailed building info from the condo board. Checking yourself would save money, but it's your call." I opted for us doing our own inspection.

"Okay Matt, keep checking things like you've been doing," Colleen said. "Be sure to check the bathroom too—sink, toilet and tub. Make sure it all works. If there's a problem, let me know." Colleen had an easy way with Matt.

Matt happily complied. We heard all the right bathroom sounds emanating from the space. The sound of gushing water told me that all taps were turned on full. I was getting fidgety, no longer able to ignore that the tub faucet kept running continuously. As I was about to excuse myself, Matt reappeared in the kitchen entryway.

"Sorry Colleen—got a problem. I can't get the bath water to shut off and the tub's filling up fast. But I definitely didn't do anything wrong."

The faucet was stripped. We had no tools, the tub was over half full and there was no on-site building manager. Everyone had visions of the tub overflowing into the suite and lobby below.

Neil raced home against all odds of retrieving a tool in time. I reassured a horror-stricken Matt that nobody blamed him. Remaining calm, Colleen wrote down that fixing the faucet by a professional plumber would be a condition of the sale. But it was Kate who casually assessed the situation and identified an interim solution.

"Let's switch the lever from tub to shower. That'll reduce water flow, which should allow the tub to drain a bit. Minimally it buys Dad time to hustle back." We all stood back and watched with relief as the water level slowly subsided.

With tragedy averted, the sale was negotiated and our elusive dream of home ownership realized. One giant leap forward.

Chapter 32: Far from Alone

Initially blinded by the unknown, we craved direction. New to parenthood and lost in a harsh, barren social landscape, concerns mounted about our young son's developmental delays. Before questions were fully formed in our brains, Neil and I were desperate for guideposts on this new and unexplored terrain. In hindsight, it was a gift that professional answers came slowly. It allowed us to gradually develop parental knowledge and confidence. We applauded our son's potential, based on lived experience, refusing to be deflated by statistical probabilities. Yet, guidance and nourishment were initially in short supply.

The inukshuk, a symbol of Canada's north, serves as a landmark to aid in navigation for its Inuit population. It also marks food caches—a vital resource if the hunting or fishing is poor. Built to resemble humans, inukshuks have been widely adopted as a symbol today, reminding people of our dependence on each other and the value of strong relationships. Like the inukshuk, advocacy represents safety, hope and guidance to those in need. Over time, we found opportunities to drink from deep streams of advocacy and share our learning with other travellers.

Invaluable diagnostic expertise, insights and professional advice played critical roles in understanding the big picture of vulnerability—both the broad sweep of the landscape, as well as its essential details. However, just as valuable was the knowledge and insights that came from lived experience—a family's emotional investment in creating a fulfilling life for one of its own.

Families lead in protecting vulnerable loved ones, yet credibility and power is heavily weighted towards professional expertise. Highly organized bureaucracies such as government social agencies tend toward the intellectual and abstract, rather than the personal. Formal credentials and titles can overshadow real-life experience with disability. Advocacy is the best strategy to help combat the inherent imbalance.

Creating networks of like-minded citizens, activists and mentors nourish families on arduous quests across this unpredictable landscape. Such connections shield and strengthen families with the knowledge that others understand and stand with them. Developing an advocacy network often starts small, as does any craftsman's set of tools.

Most navigators start with the basics—a compass, a star chart, or in these days, assistance from GPS. As with any skilled craftsmen, parents learn to maintain their tools, expand their collection and refine their skills. Master craftsmen know when and how to strategically use specific tools with precision accuracy.

Feeling worthy and having the skills to stand up for oneself is important for all citizens. Much like a personal reserve tank, resilience is essential to survive the inevitable droughts of understanding created by bureaucratic thinking. Bureaucratic systems, like any resource-rich ecosystem, ensure plenty of fuel in their reserve tanks.

Having an advocacy toolbox at one's disposal is critical for every family member, including its most vulnerable member. Ever confident, Matt has developed strong self-advocacy skills. We have first-hand experience being on the receiving end of Matt's self-advocacy. He can be a skilled swordsman in his own right.

Many self-advocates with developmental disabilities connect with the *People First* movement. The name says it all. Established in the early 1970s, the movement initially focused on closing institutions for people with developmental disabilities. Almost 50 years later, remnants of the extended institutional era still exist in Canada.

With large institutions officially eradicated, their community-based incarnation—group homes—still abound. The mentality of segregation is hard to shake for fearful families married to the concept of safety.

As our family's first foray into supported independent living revealed, superficially rebranding group-home mentality is easy. Yet

314

deeply entrenched beliefs and practices join forces whenever corporate culture is challenged. People, rather than systems, pay the price in the battle for ordinary lives. Every warrior angel needs to be armed with clarity, determination, adaptability and resilience. Only by cultivating these traits is there a chance of breaking through the protective armour of massive systems.

Some elderly parents without succession plans worry about dying. The fear's not for themselves but for the fate of their vulnerable loved one left behind. If nobody is available to assume the hefty mantle of advocate, the system will fill the void with its standardized recipe for "care." Retirement from lifelong advocacy is not an option.

As age brings deep wisdom, vitality wanes. Neil and I have learned to fall back and let others lead, like geese flying in formation. That's only possible because of a trusted advocacy network—family and others who care deeply enough to take the helm, in varying situations. Matt's support network is primarily, but not solely, cross-generational. Matt has unconditional warrior angels in his parents, sister, brother-in-law and cousin. His spirited young nieces will undoubtedly learn to wield the sword and shield.

Advocates learn to sniff the air for incongruities of words with underlying intent. The goal is promoting understanding and negotiation over battle, when possible. My stories are unique to our family yet identify recurring themes, recognized by all advocates. Every quest for ordinary lives of belonging unfolds differently, yet universally we rely on the same glue to bind and repair. Recent examples from friends in Canada, the United States and Australia reinforce this.

Holly's adult daughter, Ivy, completed an inclusive post-secondary college program in Edmonton. She has become recognized as a gifted artist. Near graduation, curious people in the disability field asked Holly if her daughter would now attend a local recreational art program for adults with developmental disabilities. Rather than seeing Ivy as an artist with a disability, they saw her disability and then looked for an art program that catered to this marginalized population. Ivy has had successful art showings and pop-up events at the university, as well as a solo exhibit at her community public library. Professional business and art mentors became actively engaged, offering marketing expertise and art advice. Most importantly, they welcomed Ivy into their respective professional communities.

Alyssa, an incredibly gifted, calm and clear communicator, teaches internationally, advocating for inclusion. Even with her highly refined skills navigating systems, challenges arose when seeking appropriate support for her adult daughter, Jasmine.

Alyssa shared her frustration about their administrative gatekeeper. "Funny that her name is Ms. Fowler. It's apt because she can be counted on to foul things up for our family every time."

Poppy, an Australian beacon of hope and inspiration for families, shares her wisdom and creativity across continents. Years of perseverance and effort evolved into personalized, rewarding and effective strategies that support her adult son. Darren, who lives with layers of complexity, experiences the richness of an ordinary life. Following a protracted review of her son's innovative, long-standing and stable living arrangement, bureaucrats proposed scrapping it, to trial a new approach. From a narrow professional perspective, the proposal sounded worth a try. The system had nothing to lose. The family on the other hand....

The family's intricate, beautifully designed creation was at high risk of collapse. Holes in the proposed government plan would quickly destabilize the carefully constructed masterpiece. The government's plan struck like an earthquake, sending shockwaves coursing through Darren's support network. What the worker perceived as good news struck terror in my friend's heart—literally. Poppy was hospitalized. The admitting doctor believed she was having a heart attack.

So how do families learn about resources and groups? Minimally, the internet is an invaluable resource. I was privileged to have multiple opportunities to participate in workshops with international inclusion gurus. Dr. Wolf Wolfensberger, John McKnight, John O'Brien, Michael Kendrick, Darcy Elks, Judith Snow, Jack Pearpoint and many more incredible advocates. They all shared deep wells of knowledge about what is, what could be, and pitfalls in the middle. Their collective wisdom and common themes gave me the courage to seek the elements of an ordinary life for our son. I'd highly recommend a Google search of these names, adding the word "inclusion." It'll lead you to a wealth of articles, videos and other resources promoting ordinary lives for marginalized populations. Powerful examples of what can be achieved and how fuels determined warrior angels around the world.

Everyone mentioned above acknowledges the foundation laid by the late Dr. Wolf Wolfensberger's large body of work. His book, the *Principle of Normalization in Human Services,* led to the Social Role Valorization (SRV) theory. SRV focuses on the importance of helping marginalized people improve their social image and attain typically valued citizenship roles—the pathway to a decent life. Next, he developed PASSING, an evaluation tool for analyzing the quality of human services. The extensive evaluation tool rates how well practices enhance the image and competency of the people served, in ways that shape ordinary lives. The tool's beauty is that it measures not in relation to system standards, but in everyday ways that align with community norms.

I highly recommend the website www.wolfwolfensberger.com, especially the header *Life's Work.* This information includes enlightening and interconnected explanations of *Normalization, SRV, Citizen Advocacy and PASSING.*

I fondly recall Dr. Wolfensberger's fascination with etymology—the root words of language. He noted that the Latin root of "client" references being carried on one's back—a burden. Not much has changed in the world of professional care since the word was first coined in ancient times. The impact is amplified when applied to those who lack valued social roles in society. Carelessly tossed barbed terms have inordinate power to taunt, diminish and ignore societal outliers. Sadly, this often goes dismissed by the privileged majority.

Michael Kendrick wondrously straddles the spectrum of government and non-government organizations. With surgical precision he dissects key issues and challenges that impact the lives of disadvantaged populations, then identifies ways forward. Adamant about the natural authority of families, his messages can reassure families when dealing with bureaucracies. Systems increasingly focus on legal authority and react to being questioned. Our son's offended public trustee is one minor example. As Michael reminds us, nobody begs for their caseworker when in anguish— their cry is for family.

Safeguards against societal exploitation and system oppression are never a guarantee for those who are marginalized. Some rare people with significant disabilities are recognized societally for excelling in some area of their life, yet they too are not exempt. Once they step outside of that valued social role, marginalization awaits.

Under the skilled tutelage of Darcy Elks, I learned Social Role Valorization theory, took intensive PASSING training and evaluated human service organizations using SRV principles. Well-intentioned staff members proudly shared agency practices, while I adopted my best poker face. How could they presume to advocate if they didn't understand the importance of looking through the lens of normal? I'd like to say the landscape has become significantly less challenging, but over decades I've not seen enduring system-wide change. While there are some fine examples of advocacy organizations and service providers helping clients achieve quality of life as citizens, they are more the exception than the norm.

If "clients" only experience living under house rules they often lack the knowledge of ordinary life to recognize the discrepancy between their life and that of typical citizens. My final career role was supervising approved *Quality of Life* interview processes across Alberta. I poignantly recall a man casually mentioning that he'd been attending the same facility weekdays for over 50 years.

The man started school at age six, in the early days of "special education." Segregated schools became the first public education program available to children with developmental disabilities. This societal recognition that they could learn was achieved through tenacious family advocacy. Access to any public education was a monumental accomplishment at the time. Decades later, the school was revamped as an adult day program facility. The segregation mill didn't skip a beat, nor did the man miss a day.

Living a counterfeit existence and shielded from ordinary living, his human capacity went untested and potential withered. This man's parents were likely warrior angels in their time, demanding and seizing a public education for their son. In current times, warrior angels demand access to the fullness of an ordinary life, stretching beyond patronization and institutional control.

My career, despite being predominantly aligned with my values, left me sceptical. Even with good consultation and planning, enactment of innovative approaches can readily get hijacked and rationalized. An example is the adoption of regional guidelines that violated provincial Principles for Determining Individual Support Needs—principles rooted in what families and individuals told the system.

Systems function best within formulas, measuring needs and calculating a budget, using standardized models of "care." In real life, formulas work for numbers, not people. The needs of people are fluid and messy. Human service systems are by nature risk-aversive, so focus on playing it safe. A life rooted in safety and security represents the road to oblivion, where mere existence and compliance are deemed markers of success. The uniqueness of each person's needs is the first casualty when systems evaluate service provision effectiveness. It's done in the name of fairness, being realistic and accountability…from the system's perspective. The antidote to systemic formulas is active citizenship, infused with advocacy and collaboration.

Families can easily be convinced they should be grateful for a life less than ordinary, measured by non-community standards and nonsensical logic that might work for widgets, not people. System arguments fall apart when we acknowledge that every person is unique and plan accordingly. Families' lived experiences put them in a far better position to identify effective approaches that bring out the best in their loved one. Michael Kendrick encourages families to be *sensibly unrealistic* when dealing with systems. It's the hidden pathway to a better, natural life. And what fuels the advocate's reserve tank? It's nourishment from each other's courage, tenacity and wisdom.

The goal for all people should be to thrive, not just survive. Advocates accept life's currents and caress our loved ones like small precious stones, while standing in the nourishing stream. With a blend of bravery and trepidation, each marginalized person's unique vulnerabilities are dropped into the mix, just like yours and mine. Every splash displaces water, creating intriguing circles, with potentially far-reaching impact. Gravity welcomes each stone to the riverbed.

Riverbeds are amazing because of their collective beauty—all sizes, shapes and colours—with each stone being distinct. The true beauty of each is revealed only after it is washed, tumbled and smoothed by life's journey. Nestled together in the riverbed of community, committed families rejoice in the wondrous elixir of ordinary life. In this fluid, ever-changing environment our son's potential has been given the opportunity to be unleashed. Life's waters have gradually smoothed his jagged edges. Come to think of it, my edges too.

Chapter 33: Nurturing *Better*

We chose to never settle. Doing so offered no solace. Seeking a life of citizenship for Matthew meant venturing into life's deep waters, with exposure to undertows and rough seas, far beyond the supposedly safe cove of clienthood. Our family minimized risks in wild storms by investing in safety equipment, waterproof gear and navigational instruments that steered us towards a land of opportunity. As all seasoned sailors know, even then we risked being shipwrecked or worse. Yet who can't relate to arduous times in their own life's quest for *better*?

Professionals are taught to keep their distance, adhere to system rules and not get personally involved—all measures that protect them from emotional involvement. Families, however, are deeply emotionally involved. As such we learn to self-nurture in the world that professionals run from. When the label of disability is slapped on people, simplistic long-term solutions of "care" routinely get dangled—problem solved. In reality it's societal attitudes, not the labelled person, that's the problem.

The gruelling quest for ordinary embodies risks, battles, leaps of faith, respect, dialogue, perseverance and vigilance. And I have an open ticket. My ride ends when I die or my faculties take an early leave. Safeguarding, while respecting Matt's adulthood and self-determination, remains a delicate balance. As Mum it wears me out. How can I do *better* when feeling like a thin overused washcloth, one day away from the rag pile?

I possess a warrior angel's spirit, but a sole warrior is not an army. I've recruited other warriors who value our son's worth. Rather than perish alone on the battlefield, I've learned to take reprieves. Others step up to respond. Challenges may still await me after I'm rested and nourished. More often these days, it gets resolved during my reprieve.

No longer the designated leader, I consult and connect with devoted warrior angels who are prepared to battle and pay the price—family and allies all. Matt's better able to navigate his world knowing these people care deeply and can be trusted to have his back. Who Matt chooses to engage with and when is up to him—all part of living life as an adult, not a man-child.

Everyone's patience has been tested, not always because of systems. Sometimes Matt's the creator of his sticky situations. Impulsiveness and *Matt logic* lead the charge, with unanticipated consequences—at least from Matt's perspective. Those who stand by him routinely remind ourselves that Matt's layers of complexity cloud his navigational skills. That context helps us better understand when, why and how to hold Matt accountable. It also implores us to assess our personal role in doing better.

Officially a senior citizen, I exuded excellent health, until the day I didn't. Mere days before Christmas 2016, a grand mal seizure shocked everyone, especially me. Extensive neurological testing and a medication rollercoaster marked the first year. Insidious emotional and physical challenges hopped aboard too. Stamina plummeted. Tenacious by nature, it took a long time to admit that determination alone wouldn't fix things. Neil, Kate and Matt worried about small fractures in my shield, ones that eluded me initially.

No answers were ever found, life stabilized and I became accepting of this slightly altered me. With a twinkle in his eye, Neil contests that it's more than *slightly*. While he does have a point, the bottom line is that I'm still me and will always push myself to do better. My capacity to juggle multiple responsibilities, projects and unexpected challenges while keeping stress at bay is diminished, but manageable—at least on most days. It requires ongoing self-monitoring and heeding telltale warning signs of *too much*. Forever a challenge.

My initial post-trauma year gave me a glimpse into how Matt experiences the world. I struggled to perform and multitask daily life. I needed bite-size morsels in order to process large amounts of information. Off balance, both physically and emotionally, I questioned things. Not because I doubted information being shared, but to ensure I understood correctly. Questioning sometimes tested the patience of people who love me. This distressing experience, my blip in time, reflects ongoing life for Matt.

This gem of wisdom that was dropped into my hands can readily slip through fingers—firmly grasped intellectually until human emotions trigger its release. Intellect and emotions are becoming better aligned, but are never guaranteed. When tired, it's easy to snap first and step back later. Neil gently reminds me to be a realist with our son, noting that harping doesn't work.

Family relationships have become more balanced—bringing comfort and rewards. For years Matt turned to me for information, guidance and solace. Relatively recently, Matt's begun engaging Neil and it's opened up a communication stream that was dammed far too long. Matt routinely seeks Neil's input on medical and technological matters. Neil shrugs his shoulders, minimizing the extent of his knowledge, yet it impresses both Matt and me. Matt's confiding in Kate far more frequently too. Besides nurturing his role as the doting uncle, he seeks and increasingly listens to sibling input about relationships, financial considerations and practical condo matters that need attention.

During a recent phone call from Kate, her voice danced with amusement. "So, I hear you're mad at Matt."

"So mad I could spit! Trading his prized brand-new television—for a laptop—*supposedly* so he can submit resumes. It's his damn impulsivity, plain and simple! So proud of saving for that TV and swore he'd never get rid of it. That lasted what—maybe two weeks?" My tirade vented some excess frustration.

"Sounds about right. Mum, we all know how he can't resist when something jumps out as a 'better deal.' But he's desperate to make amends with you by returning the laptop and getting the TV back. A small hitch—he spent the difference so is a *bit* short." She tittered and continued. "Not surprising. Although the TV was better, he can still watch shows on the laptop. So is it really a big deal?"

"Think about his history, Kate. Within a week he'll convince himself that it's fine to take the laptop on the bus. Experience shows that he'll likely lose it, panic, stress and have no entertainment at home."

"Shoot—you're absolutely right! Let's make a plan to help him get his TV back." So together, with Matt's input, we did.

Matt typically misses the point when I get frustrated over mundane things. In all likelihood, he always will. What he doesn't recognize is that all those little things pile high like playing a game of pick-up-sticks. Each one is carefully assessed and extracted with jubilation, until the pile shifts. That ends the game. I'm done and he's bewildered. Later in the week, I'll likely give him the same suggestion. The sender and receiver roles change frequently—it's just part of our reality.

"But I love you, Mum…."

That truth always makes me want to stick a dagger in my heart. I've worked hard to remind myself that I have the capacity to see the big picture, identifying and implementing strategies for *me* to do better, not Matt. The chances of our son doing better increase when he feels understood and valued. That's what allows him to hear and potentially absorb my message. Nagging and non-verbal communication, like sighs and eye rolling, reinforce society's message that *he's* not good enough.

Although committed to recalibrating my compass, it's not uncommon to slip up. I don't handle things well when weary of the frequent reach outs or *Matt logic* dilemmas.

"Hello, again," I sigh. "Matt you've called me at least 10 times already today." Then with a hint of annoyance, "What's up *now?*"

"Don't think it's been that many times. Maybe five…no, just four, I think. Forget why I was calling. Probably 'cause I love you guys and miss you a lot. Sure enjoyed my visit out there last time."

"Matt, I love you too but please don't call so often. I'm doing laundry and housework, same as when you called an hour ago. Maybe good things for you to do."

"Thank you!" he shouted.

"Huh—for what?"

"Oh, not you. Just thanking the bus driver. Almost home now. What were you saying, Mum?"

"Not much. Talk to you tomorrow." After hanging up, I stand and stare out the window.

Gazing across the lake at the majestic mountain view helps relieve tension in my mind and body. It doesn't matter if it's a blue sky day or gloomy with clouds skimming the water. The rugged mountains embody beauty, uncertainty, imposing terrain, surprises and risks. All traits that reflect a life well lived. I begin to breathe easier.

Exercising regularly with karate and yoga help with fitness and life balance. Engagement in refreshingly abundant social opportunities and volunteering round out my days. At this stage of life, I'm past taking things on from a sense of obligation. Being true to myself allows me to live my best life.

Choosing to retire in a small village, a full 10-hour drive away from Matt, was not a decision made lightly. But like Matt, we deserve a life of possibility, opportunity and fulfillment. We accomplished it by nurturing long-term relationships, putting safeguards in place and fostering Matt's capacity to do *better*, without parents hovering around. And the phone puts us in ready contact with Matt and those who support him. Enhanced understanding and responsiveness to our most vulnerable member's realities nourishes family connectedness and strengthens our humanity.

Life lessons keep coming my way and Matt's often the messenger. Most battles these days are internal. Hindsight occasionally still likes to poke me. That's when I need to cradle myself—a flawed mortal,

325

living in a turbulent, complex world. It brings me comfort knowing that I didn't settle for less than a chance for Matt to live an ordinary life as a valued citizen. I may have compromised or acquiesced out of exhaustion, but never did I compromise on values and principles.

My brain unexpectedly releases a lesson from the vault of advocacy training. I'm reminded that all humans can do is celebrate the good things and problem solve the rest. That's what nurturing *better* looks like.

Snapshots from Matt's Journey

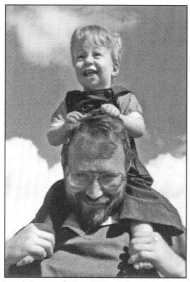

On Top of the World with Dad
Brother

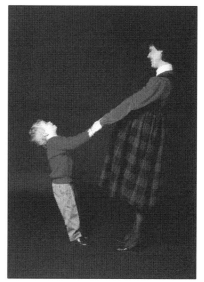

Soon to be Big

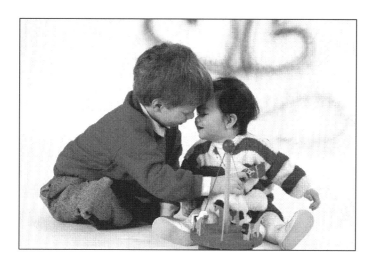

Matt & Kate Valentines

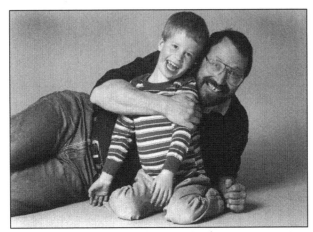

Matt & Neil United

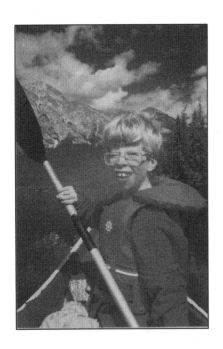

Novice Paddler

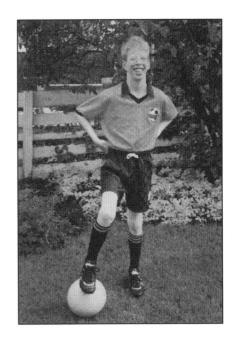

Community Soccer Player

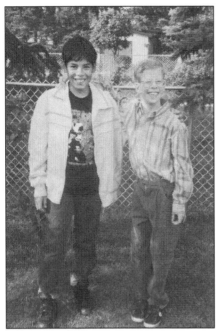

Best Friends, Matt & Gary.

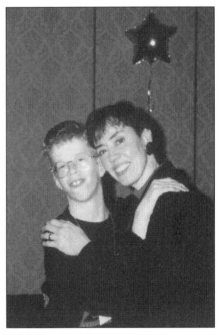

Matt and Susan at Williams Syndrome Conference

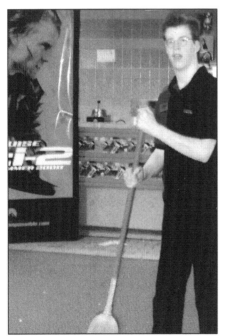

Movie Theatre Employee

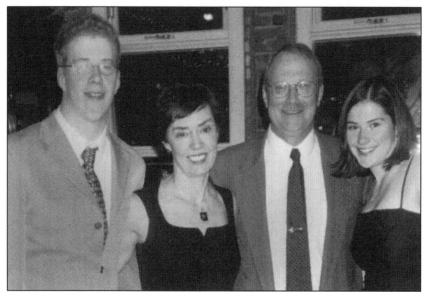

Matt, Susan, Neil & Kate

Esks #1 Fan

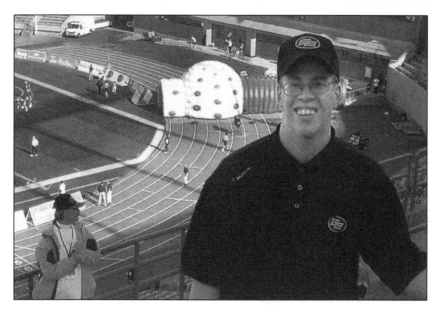

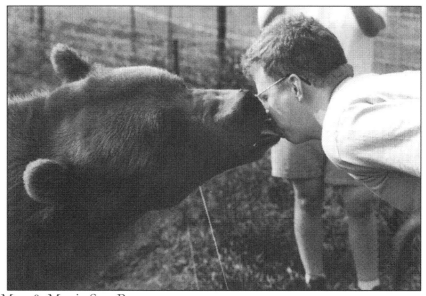

Matt & Movie Star Bear

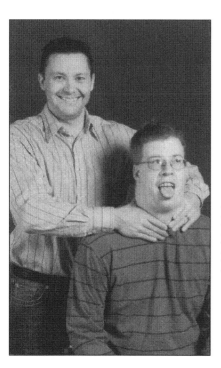

Proud
Owner of
Angelo

Like
Brothers,
Martin &
Matt

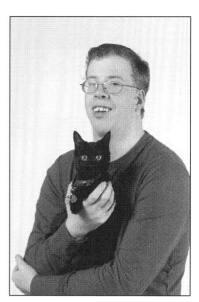

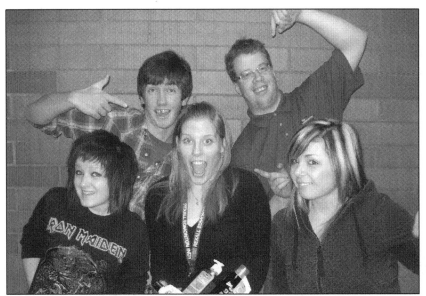

College Classmates

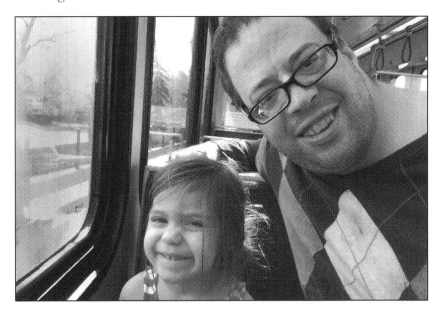

Introducing Devyn to Transit

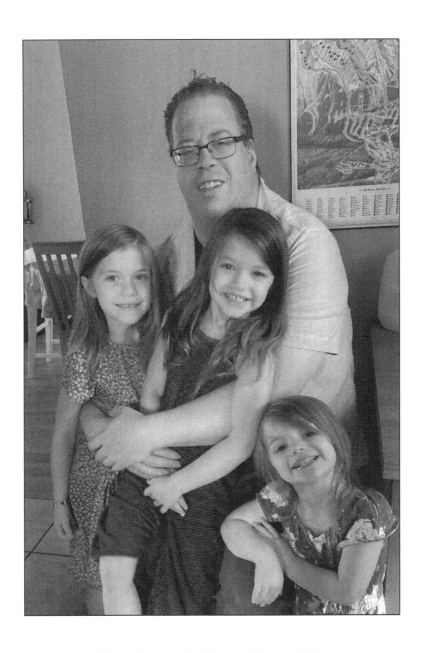

Uncle Matt with Devyn, Alex and Zoe

Conclusion

Our family's arduous quest for *ordinary* merited reflection. Relentless years of challenges, setbacks and judgement took their toll on every family member. Like all who pursue inclusion and social justice, nobody went unscathed. Garish battle scars have receded from prominence, becoming subtle badges of honour for having survived. Peace rather than battle has become more common, although skirmishes can still flare.

At times we felt alone, but truly weren't. Once connected with other passionate families and advocates, we were embraced within a larger family of the heart. Warrior angels all. Love fuelled our army. Individually we stumbled, fell, got up and retreated, into the arms of caring allies who tended to our wounds. Families' voices coalesced into one, echoing across the battlefield. Never alone.

While battles are short, intense and bloody, rebellions are protracted and speak to the bigger picture. Elusive social justice is integral to my being, residing in my heart, blood and bones. That was reflected in my career choices before the birth of our vulnerable son. Matthew became the sinew that connected all aspects of my life.

Core values have always shaped how my family lives—our moral compass. Whenever our family got knocked off course, recalibration pointed us in the right direction—far away from a life of *clienthood*.

Matt's life likely comes up short compared to most former school peers, although significant challenges undoubtedly awaited them too. We chose to honour Matt as an adult with lead responsibility for life choices—the societal norm. Those who love and respect him are available to mentor, guide and console from the sidelines. Any doubts about our path through the wilderness have long been eradicated. At times we were stuck, stung, cold, thirsty and lost. Yet perseverance drew us to meadows and streams where we drank wisdom from the cup of others. As individuals and a family, we became better human beings for having faced the wilderness and tested our mettle.

A memorabilia folder compiled from our son's youth is reflective of his journey growing up. The varied content includes letters, homework, contest entries, thank-you notes and more. Among the treasures was a collection of letters our son wrote on subjects of importance to him. Recipients included neighbours, family, classmates, local flyer supervisors, authors, senior government officials and the head of the Canadian Football League (CFL). Far-reaching topics spoke to his entrepreneurial business ventures, petitioning for someone's heart transplant, love for family, wanting a *bad call* reviewed from a CFL Grey Cup game and much more. Neil and I savour each piece of paper and the memories they conjure up. We've laughed and dabbed away brewing tears as our hearts glowed. This folder reflects Matt in his entirety—sensitivity, kindness, awareness of personal challenges and a unique approach to life.

Do I wish Matt had a fuller life? Yes. Unfortunately, in recent years, his interconnected health issues have limited viable employment options. Being without part-time employment strips him of a valued social role, while limiting his role as a consumer with disposable income. Health realities restrict, but don't rule out the prospect of meaningful work. However, finding the right match will require creative thinking and engaging with flexible, open-minded employers who are willing to accommodate. I'm convinced that such elusive opportunities are waiting to be seized. It will happen when Matt's ready and with support of those who believe in his capacity, as a citizen, not a client.

I understand the temptation of families to choose what is billed as the safer, easier route—letting bureaucrats and systems lead. Decades of professional experience from within the human services system only reaffirms my stance. While Matt's life carries elements of risk and uncertainty, that's typical of ordinary lives. *Citizenship over*

Clienthood will always be our family's mantra, as exemplified in the stories I shared.

Perfection is a myth and fallibility is a given. As eloquently stated by Winston Churchill, "Success is not final, failure is not fatal. It is the courage to continue that counts."

My cherished *Warrior Angel* sculpture epitomizes the struggle. Metaphorically, the broadsword represents the willingness to defend core values and beliefs, despite the cost. One never truly reaches mastery of the sword. Perseverance and effort hone skills and deepen one's understanding. Firmly rooted, nurtured and accepting our human imperfections strengthen resilience. It's all about striving for better, a quest that never ends. Matt and all family members embrace life in the midst of ordinary community. And that's where we all belong.

Disclaimer

Warrior Angel identifies real incidents and replicates associated dialogue, reflecting personal memories to the best of my ability. Any errors or omissions in my recollections are mine alone. Some names in the book have been changed to protect the privacy of individuals.

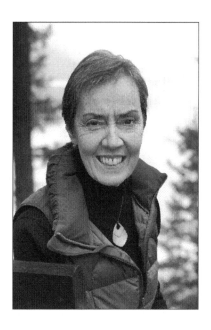

About the Author:

Trained as a social worker, parenthood solidified Susan's education. Over 35 years ago, her son's emerging disability related challenges fused personal and professional worlds. Candour, sensitivity, empathy and passion filled every crevice of both realms. Now retired, Susan worked on behalf of marginalized populations for 40 years. Half of her career was in the field of developmental disability, interweaving policy development, implementation, service delivery and accountability. The icing on the cake was her training as an advocate, fiercely focused on inclusion. A warrior angel amidst an army of compatriots.

For more information visit Susan's website at seekingordinary.com

Manufactured by Amazon.ca
Bolton, ON